A LEXICON OF LUNACY

Books by Thomas Szasz

Pain and Pleasure
The Myth of Mental Illness
Law, Liberty, and Psychiatry
Psychiatric Justice
The Ethics of Psychoanalysis
The Manufacture of Madness
Ideology and Insanity
The Age of Madness (ed.)
The Second Sin
Ceremonial Chemistry
Heresies
Karl Kraus and the Soul Doctors
Schizophrenia
Psychiatric Slavery
The Theology of Medicine
The Myth of Psychotherapy
Sex by Prescription
The Therapeutic State
Insanity
The Untamed Tongue
Our Right to Drugs
A Lexicon of Lunacy
Cruel Compassion
The Meaning of Mind
Fatal Freedom
Pharmacracy
Liberation by Oppression

A LEXICON OF LUNACY

Metaphoric Malady, Moral Responsibility, and Psychiatry

Thomas Szasz

Transaction Publishers
New Brunswick (U.S.A.) and London (U.K.)

First paperback printing 2003
Copyright © 1993 by Transaction Publishers, New Brunswick, New Jersey.

This book is printed on acid-free paper that meets the American National Standard for Permanence of Paper for Printed Library Materials.

Library of Congress Catalog Number: 92-5866
ISBN: 1-56000-065-1 (cloth); 0-7658-0506-5 (paper)
Printed in the United States of America

Library of Congress Cataloging-in-Publication Data

Szasz, Thomas Stephen, 1920-
A lexicon of lunacy : metaphoric malady, moral responsibility, and psychiatry / Thomas Szasz.
    p. cm.
 Includes bibliographical references and index.
 ISBN 0-7658-0506-5 (alk. paper)
   1. Antipsychiatry. 2. Mental health personnel—Language. 3. Mental illness—Terminology. 4. Psycholinguistics. I. Title.

RC437.5.S89 1992
616.89'001—dc20   92-5866
                                                    CIP

How easy it is to make people
believe a lie, and how hard it is
to undo that work again!
                    —Mark Twain

Contents

Preface   ix
Acknowledgments   xi
Introduction   1

I. LANGUAGE AND LUNACY

1. Shakespeare's Plays   13
2. The Contemporary Scene   21
3. Dictionaries of Deviance   37
   A. DSM-III-R Classification of Mental Disorders   40
   B. Synonyms for Mental Illness   46
   C. Synonyms for Mental Hospital   78
4. Dictionaries of Drunkenness   81
   A. Benjamin Franklin's "The Drinkers Dictionary"   83
   B. Edmund Wilson's "The Lexicon of Prohibition"   89
   C. A Contemporary Dictionary of Drunkenness   91

II. METAPHORIC MALADY, MORAL RESPONSIBILITY, AND PSYCHIATRY

5. The Religion Called "Psychiatry"   101
6. Mental Illness and Mental Incompetence   111
7. The Illusion of Mental Patients' Rights   127
8. The Illusion of Drug Abuse Treatment   143
9. The Case Against Suicide Prevention   147
10. The Psychiatric Will   159
11. *Ex Parte* Psychiatry   173
Epilogue   183
Notes   187
Index   199

Preface

Anyone with an ear for language recognizes that the line separating the seemingly serious vocabulary of psychiatric diagnosis from the ludicrous lexicon of psychobabble, and both from the jesting colloquialism of slang, is thin at best and nonexistent at worst. Therein precisely lie the beauty, the richness, and the power of language. If we want to say something tactfully that might otherwise offend, we say it, as the adage has it, in jest, but mean it in earnest. Bureaucrats, politicians, quacks, and other assorted mountebanks typically say things in earnest; but if we want to protect ourselves from being victimized by them, we had better hear their messages in jest. Anyone who takes the bad jokes of psychiatric diagnoses seriously does so at his own peril.

As in all my writings on psychiatry, I use certain phrases—such as *mental illness, psychiatric diagnosis*, and *psychiatric treatment*—whose conventional meanings I reject. To avoid defacing the text, I have refrained from putting such prejudging expressions between quotations marks each time they appear. Also, for the sake of brevity and convenience, I often use the terms *psychiatrist, patient*, and *mental hospital* to refer to mental health professionals, mental health clients, and mental health institutions of all kinds.

This book consists of two parts. Part I is a critical reflection on the extraordinary profusion of terms in American English for behaviors conventionally called "mental illnesses," together with as complete a listing of such terms as I have been able to assemble. In addition, because American English contains an amazingly large number of figures of speech for drunkenness (which have attracted the attention of students of language), and because in the United States drinking to excess is regarded as a bona fide disease, I also include here three lists of terms and phrases referring specifically to this form of behavior.

Part II is a collection of previously published papers that illustrate our propensity to use the language of mental illness to influence social relationships—in particular, to reduce or annul personal responsibility by shifting it from self to others or to the fiction of mental illness. Each of these papers has been extensively revised, some so thoroughly that they may fairly be counted as fresh essays.

Acknowledgments

Once again, I thank my daughter Suzy and brother George for their steadfast support; Roger Yanow and Charles S. Howard for their constructive criticism; and Peter Uva, librarian at the SUNY Health Science Center, for his unfailing help.

I wish to thank the following sources for permission to use the materials that appear in this volume in adapted form. Parts of the "Introduction," from "Diagnoses Are Not Diseases," *The Lancet* 338:(21/28 December 1991)1574-76; "The Religion Called 'Psychiatry,'" from "The Religion Called 'Psychiatry,'" *Second Opinion* 6 (November 1987):50-61; "Mental Illness and Mental Incompetence," from, "Illness and Incompetence," David J. Schnall and Carl L. Figliola, eds., *Contemporary Issues in Health Care* (New York: Praeger, 1984), 112-25; "The Illusion of Mental Patients' Rights," from "The Myth of the Rights of Mental Patients," *Liberty* 2(July 1989): 19-26; "The Illusion of Drug Abuse Treatment," from "The Myth of Treatment," *The Drug Policy Letter* 3(Fall 1991):3-4; "The Case Against Suicide Prevention," from, "The Case Against Suicide Prevention," *American Psychologist* 41(July 1986):806-12; "The Psychiatric Will," from, "The Psychiatric Will: A New Mechanism for Protecting Person Against 'Psychosis' and Psychiatry," *American Psychologist* 37(July 1982):762-70; "*Ex Parte* Psychiatry," from, "Psychiatric Justice," *British Journal of Psychiatry* 154(June 1989):864-69.

I also thank the following publishers for permission to reprint materials copyrighted by them: American Psychiatric Association, for the roster of diagnoses from the *Diagnostic and Statistical Manual of Mental Disorders of the American Psychiatric Association* (*DSM-III-R*), Third Edition - Revised; Charles C. Thomas, Publisher, for synonyms for *malingering*, from *Dictionary of Medical Slang and Related Esoteric Expressions*, by J. E. Schmidt; Farrar, Straus & Giroux, for "The Lexicon of Prohibition," by Edmund Wilson; Gale Research, Inc., for material from -*Ologies & -Isms*, ed. Laurence Urdang; and Oxford University Press, for partial list of phobias, from *Psychiatric Dictionary*, by R. J. Campbell.

Introduction

*Learn to recognize the symptoms of MENTAL
ILLNESS. Schizophrenia, Manic Depression and
Severe Depression are BRAIN DISEASES.*
—Hawaii State Alliance for the Mentally Ill

Intrigued by the patently metaphoric character of the psychiatric vocabulary—which, nevertheless, is widely recognized as a legitimate medical idiom—I decided, at the beginning of my professional career, to explore the nature and function of these literalized metaphors, and to expose them to public scrutiny. I thus set in motion a controversy about mental illness which is still raging, and whose essence is still often misunderstood. Many scientists, physicians, jurists, and lay persons believe that the demonstration of a genetic defect or a brain lesion in so-called mental patients would prove that mental illnesses exist and are like any other disease. This is not so. If mental illnesses are diseases of the central nervous system, then they are diseases of the brain, not the mind. And if mental illnesses are the names of (mis)behaviors, then they are behaviors, not diseases. A screwdriver may be a drink or an implement. No amount of research on orange juice and vodka can establish that it is a hitherto unrecognized form of a carpenter's tool.

Although linguistic clarification is valuable for individuals who want to think clearly, it is not useful for people whose social institutions rest on the unexamined, literal use of language. Accordingly, I have long maintained that psychiatric metaphors have the same role in our Therapeutic Society that religious metaphors have in Theological Societies. For example, there is consensus among Mohammedans that their God wants them to worship on Friday, among Jews that theirs wants them to worship on Saturday, and among Christians that theirs wants them to worship on Sunday. Similarly, the various versions of the American Psychiatric Association's *Diagnostic and Statistical Manual* rest only on consensus. Let me illustrate this contention with a simple, syllogistic example.

How does a dead person become a saint? By the Vatican's declaring him to be a saint. Thereafter, say, Peter and Paul are called "saints," and Catholics (and perhaps others as well) believe that Saint Peter and Saint Paul *are* saints.

1

How does the behavior of a living person become an illness? By the American Psychiatric Association's declaring it to be an illness. Thereafter, say, gambling or smoking are called "diseases," and psychiatrists and their followers (and perhaps others as well) believe that Pathological Gambling and Nicotine Dependence *are* diseases.

Still, if a person believes that mental illnesses are illnesses, his conviction is not likely to be dispelled by my argument. The religious character of the belief in mental illness manifests itself in another way as well. Religion is, among other things, the institutionalized denial of the human foundations of meaning and of the inevitable finiteness of life; the person who seeks transcendental meaning and rejects the reality of death can thus theologize life and entrust its management to clerical professionals. Likewise, psychiatry is, among other things, the institutionalized denial of the reality of free will and of the tragic nature of life; individuals who seek impersonal explanations of horrifying human action and reject the inevitability of personal responsibility can thus medicalize life and entrust its management to health professionals. Marx was close to the mark when he asserted that "Religion is the opiate of the people." But religion is not the opiate of the people; the human mind is. After all, religion is a product of our own minds, and so, too, is psychiatry. In short, the mind is its own opiate. And its ultimate drug is the Word.

Indeed, Freud himself flirted with such a formulation, but backed away from its implications, preferring instead to believe that "neuroses" are literal diseases, and that "psychoanalysis" is a literal treatment—in fact, the best treatment for these ostensibly genuine maladies. In his essay "Psychical (or Mental) Treatment," Freud wrote:

> Foremost among such measures [which operate upon the human mind] is the use of words; and words are the essential tool of mental treatment. A layman will no doubt find it hard to understand how pathological disorders of the body and mind can be eliminated by 'mere' words. He will feel that he is being asked to believe in magic. And he will not be so very wrong. . . . But we shall have to follow a roundabout path in order to explain how science sets about restoring to words a part at least of their former magical power.[1]

Despite this historical background and these epistemological considerations, an editorial in the prestigious British medical magazine *The Lancet* remains fixated on the mirage of finding the cause of schizophrenia in the brain. Lamenting the state of psychiatry 150 years after the founding of the (British) Association of Medical Officers of Asylums and

Hospitals for the Insane—today, the Royal College of Psychiatrists—the editorial writer commented:

> What about psychiatric research? We seem to be no closer to finding the real, presumed biological, causes of the major psychiatric illnesses. This is not to decry the value of such research—if the causes of conditions such as . . . schizophrenia are found it will be an advance of the same magnitude as the identification of the syphilis spirochaete in the brains of patients with general paralysis of the insane.[2]

I took up the profession of psychiatry in part to debunk the biological-reductionist impulse that has motivated its very origin and that continues to fuel its engines; in other words, to combat the contention that abnormal behaviors must be understood as the products of abnormal brains. Ironically, it was easier to do this nearly half a century ago than today. For three centuries, the idea that every "mental illness" will prove to be a bona fide brain disease was a hypothesis that could be supported or opposed. However, after the 1960s, this hypothesis became increasingly accepted as a scientific fact. Of course, it is still possible to say that mental illnesses do not exist. But since only a charlatan, a fool, or a fanatic disputes facts or opposes science, such a critic is likely to be dismissed as irrational, or worse.

Thus, for the time being at least, psychiatrists and their powerful allies have succeeded in persuading the scientific community, the courts, the media, and the general public that the conditions they call "mental disorders" are diseases—that is, phenomena independent of human motivation or will. This is a curious development, for, until recently, only psychiatrists—who know little about medicine and less about science—embraced such blind physical reductionism. Most scientists knew better. Michael Polanyi wrote:

> We can see then that, though rooted in the body, the mind is free in its actions—exactly as our common sense knows it to be free. The mind harnesses neurophysiological mechanisms; though it depends on them, it is not determined by them.[3]

Polanyi emphasized that a scientist does not make grandiose theoretical claims or flamboyant promises of impending therapeutic triumphs, but accepts certain limitations and builds on the possible:

> The recognition of certain basic impossibilities has laid the foundations of some major principles of physics and chemistry; similarly, recognition of the impossibility of understanding living things in terms of physics and chemistry, far from setting limits to our understanding of life, will guide it in the right direction.[4]

It is not by accident that the more firmly psychiatrically-inspired ideas take hold of the collective American mind, the more foolishness and injustice they generate. The Americans With Disabilities Act (AWDA), a federal law enacted in 1990 and scheduled to be fully implemented by July 1992, is an example.

The aim of the law, in part, is "to diminish the stigma of mental illness and reduce discrimination involving . . . at least 60 million Americans, between the ages of 18 and 64, [who] will experience a mental disorder during their lifetimes."[5] If this is the politically and psychiatrically correct view, how can I maintain that there are no mental disorders? Not very easily. But then, Will Rogers can be summoned for help. "Compared to those fellows in Congress," he wrote, "I'm just an amateur . . . [E]very time they make a joke, it's a law! and every time they make a law, it's a joke."[6] The AWDA is a law, but that does not prevent it from being a joke—and a very bad one at that.

Long ago, our lawmakers acquiesced in letting psychiatrists literalize the metaphor of mental illness. Having embraced "mental diseases," they now had to identify which of these manufactured maladies were covered, and which were not covered, under the AWDA. They did so by creating a list of congressionally accredited mental diseases. The AWDA covers "claustrophobia, personality problems, and mental retardation, [but does not cover] kleptomania, pyromania, compulsive gambling, and . . . transvestism."[7] At least Congress agrees with me that stealing, setting fires, gambling, and cross dressing are not diseases. But it is positively comical that our senators and congressmen do not realize that they have no more ground for excluding these alleged disorders from AWDA coverage, than they have for including those that they accept for coverage.

At about the same time as these reports on a "New Deal for the Mentally Ill" appeared in the press,[8] the *American Journal of Psychiatry* (the American Psychiatric Association's official journal) published an article on kleptomania.[9] In keeping with the *DSM-III-R* (the revised edition of *DSM-III*), the author's premise was that kleptomania is a genuine illness. His conclusion was to propose "a biopsychosocial model of the *etiology* of kleptomania . . . [which] emphasizes possible childhood abuse as a precipitating factor . . ."[10] However, the American Psychiatric Association recognizes claustrophobia (which the AWDA accepts as a mental illness) and kleptomania (which the AWDA rejects) as mental disorders on equal footing.

I will not discuss here what is meant by the word *disease*. Suffice it to say that we do not attribute motives to diseases, and do not call motivated actions (bodily) "diseases." For instance, we attribute no motive to a person for having leukemia; it would be foolish to say that a particular motive led to a person's having glaucoma; and it would be absurd to assert that an illness (say, diabetes) caused a person to become a senator. In short, one of the most important political-philosophical features of the concept of mental illness is that, at one fell swoop, it removes motivation from action, adds it to illness, and thus destroys the very possibility of distinguishing disease from nondisease.[11] This crucial function of the idea of mental illness is illustrated by the psychiatrists' classifying certain cases of theft as a disease (kleptomania), by the media's acceptance of this behavior as a disease, and by the mental health professionals' accounts of its alleged causes.

In a newspaper report on shoplifting, the director of Onondaga (New York) County's Drinking and Driving Program explains: "Syracuse needs Shoplifters Anonymous . . . There are more than 3,000 arrests for shoplifting in Onondaga County. It's costing everyone a fortune."[12] Although the program is described as "voluntary," it is a substitute for a criminal penalty: "If the thief completes the course, the arrest vanishes from his or her record." The report shows that both so-called experts and the media treat shoplifting as a disease, to which they then nevertheless attribute various motives. In the treatment program, the shoplifters "learn *why* they steal . . . there are several reasons why people shoplift. They feel entitled. Perhaps they feel prices are too high; they are angry at authority . . . It's a mental health problem."[13]

Another article describes "shopping addiction . . . as a situation where a person may utilize shopping as an activity to change their [sic] mood."[14] Such a person "really doesn't like shopping. It's not a free experience, because it has a very driven quality to it." The experts cited in this piece do not even pretend to present pathological (anatomic or physiological) evidence to support their claim; instead, they drop the names of "famous addicted shoppers . . . [such as] Princess Diana, Jacqueline Kennedy Onassis, and Imelda Marcos," ostensibly as proof that "shopaholism" is a disease. Is addiction to shopping "treatable?" the reporter inquires.

"Yes, but with variable results, say the experts. . . . The treatment is very much like any other addiction . . . you have to look at it as a life-long process."[15] *Cui bono*?

Although Congress has so far remained unconvinced that the behavior psychiatrists call kleptomania, but that most people still call shoplifting, is a genuine illness, it might be of interest to list here a few of the behaviors for which psychiatrists have disease names and that the AWDA implicitly accepts as genuine diseases, on equal footing with, say, malaria and melanoma:

300.70 BODY DYSMORPHIC DISORDER (DYSMORPHOPHOBIA). The essential feature of this disorder is preoccupation with some imagined defect in appearance in a normal-appearing person.[16]

300.14 MULTIPLE PERSONALITY DISORDER. The essential feature of this disorder is the existence within the person of two or more distinct personalities. . . . At least two of the personalities, at some time and recurrently, take full control of the person's behavior.[17]

302.89 FROTTEURISM. The essential feature of this disorder is recurrent, intense, sexual urges and sexually arousing fantasies, of at least six months' duration, involving touching and rubbing against a nonconsenting person.[18]

302.71 HYPOACTIVE SEXUAL DESIRE DISORDER. Persistently or recurrently deficient or absent sexual fantasies and desire for sexual activity. The judgment of deficiency or absence is made by the clinician.[19]

301.51 FACTITIOUS DISORDER WITH PHYSICAL SYMPTOMS. The essential feature of this disorder is the intentional production of physical symptoms. The presentation may be a total fabrication, as in complaints of acute abdominal pain in the absence of any such pain.[20]

The political and popular acceptance of such and similar psychiatric words and phrases as medical terms identifying genuine diseases generates a steady stream of absurd situations. But because we judge psychiatric dispositions to be humane, neither the erroneous nature of psychiatric premises nor the injustice of psychiatric dispositions discredits psychiatry as a medical specialty. The following case history serves as a good example.

A forty-two-year-old, female orthopedic surgeon, working in a Virginia suburb of Washington, D. C., is arrested for drunken driving. She resists arrest, refuses to take a breath or blood test, curses and kicks the police. Taken into custody, she finally consents to take a breath test and registers 0.13 g/dL, over the 0.10 g/dL legal limit for blood alcohol. "At trial she maintained that the circumstances of her behavior at the time of her arrest were a result of PMS [premenstrual syndrome]." She was acquitted.[21]

Psychiatric News (the American Psychiatric Association's biweekly newspaper) asked: "Does LLPDD [late luteal phase dysphoric disorder] exist?" The same question might be raised about every nonbodily disease. The reporter then cites the comments of several psychiatrists that dramatically show psychiatry's intellectual bankruptcy and moral desolation: "The decision as to whether or not LLPDD will be assigned its own diagnostic category in the fourth edition of the APA's *Diagnostic and Statistical Manual of Mental Disorders (DSM-IV)* is 'a political land mine,' according to Allen Frances, M.D., chair of the Task Force on *DSM-IV*."[22] David Rubinow, M.D., a psychiatrist who "has done research at NIH on PMS for more than a decade," offered this opinion: "As far as I am concerned, the decision to include PMS in *DSM-IV* will be made on political rather than medical considerations . . . It's quite clear there are a substantial number of people with PMS who never get arrested. To attribute guilt in a crime to PMS is a somewhat hazardous enterprise."[23]

The same argument can be made about any mental illness used to support an insanity defense. John W. Hinckley, Jr. was acquitted of shooting President Reagan because psychiatrists testified he had schizophrenia. But how many people diagnosed as schizophrenic shoot a president? And of those who do, how many claim they did it to impress Jody Foster? Actually, Hinckley's act was a unique performance that, in some ways, may be more revealing of the actor's character than his ordinary behaviors, performed routinely. Understandably, psychiatrists deny this. They realize that their entire enterprise hinges on society's acceptance of the proposition that human beings diagnosed as mentally ill have a brain disease that deprives them of free will.

Before concluding these introductory remarks, I want to say a few words about the differences between diseases and diagnoses. Diseases (in the literal sense of the term), like avalanches or earthquakes, occur naturally; whereas diagnoses, like books or bridges, are artifacts. Which raises the question: Why do we make diagnoses? There are several reasons:

1. Scientific—to identify the organs or tissues affected and perhaps the cause of the illness.

2. Professional—to enlarge the scope, and thus the power and prestige, of a state-protected medical monopoly and the income of its practitioners.

3. Legal—to justify state-sanctioned coercive interventions outside of the criminal justice system.

4. Social-economic—to authenticate persons as legitimate occupants of the sick role: for example, to secure drugs, compensation payments, etc. available only to bona fide sick (diagnosed) patients.

5. Political-economic—to justify enacting and enforcing measures aimed at promoting public health and providing funds for research and treatment on projects classified as medical.

6. Personal—to enlist the support of public opinion, the media, and the legal system for bestowing special privileges (and impose special penalties) on persons diagnosed as (mentally) ill.

It is not coincidence that most psychiatric diagnoses are twentieth-century inventions. The aim of the classic, nineteenth-century model of diagnosis was to identify bodily lesions (diseases) and their material causes (etiology). For example, the term *pneumococcal pneumonia*—a paradigm of a pathology-driven diagnosis—identifies the organ affected, the lungs, and the cause of the illness, infection with the pneumococcus.[24] Diagnoses driven by other motives—such as the desire to coerce the patient or to secure government funding for the treatment of his (alleged) illness—generate different diagnostic constructions, and lead to different conceptions of disease.

Today, even diagnoses of what were strictly medical diseases are no longer pathology-driven. The diagnoses of patients with illnesses such as asthma or arthritis, and of those requiring surgical interventions, are distorted by economic factors (especially third-party funding of hospital costs and physicians' fees). Final diagnoses on the discharge summaries of hospitalized patients are often no longer made by physicians, but by bureaucrats skilled in the ways of Medicare, Medicaid, and private health insurance reimbursement (based partly on what ails the patient, and partly on which medical terms for his ailment and treatment ensure the most generous compensation for the services rendered).[25]

In short, no psychiatric diagnosis is, or can be, pathology-driven; instead, all such diagnoses are driven by nonmedical (economic, personal, legal, political, and social) factors or incentives. Accordingly, psychiatric diagnoses do not point to pathoanatomic or pathophysiological lesions and do not identify causative agents—but refer rather to *human behaviors*. Moreover, the psychiatric terms used to refer to such behaviors allude to the plight of the denominated patient, hint at the dilemmas with which patient and psychiatrist alike try to cope as well as exploit, and mirror the beliefs and values of the society that both inhabit.

Despite their misleading—indeed, mendacious, titles—the various versions of the APA's *Diagnostic and Statistical Manual of Mental Disorders* are not classifications of mental disorders (or diseases or conditions of any kind) that "patients have." Instead, they are rosters of psychiatric diagnoses officially accredited as mental diseases by the APA.[26] This is why in psychiatry, unlike in the rest of medicine, the members of "consensus groups" and "task forces," appointed by officers of the association, make and unmake psychiatric diagnoses; and sometimes the entire membership votes on whether a controversial diagnosis is or is not a disease. For more than a century, psychiatrists created diagnoses and pretended they were diseases—and no one in authority challenged their deception. It is not surprising, then, that few people now realize that diagnoses are not diseases.[27]

I

LANGUAGE AND LUNACY

1

Shakespeare's Plays

Let us consider Shakespeare's masterpiece, Ham-
*let . . . It was not until the material of the tragedy
had been traced back by psychoanalysis to the
Oedipus theme, that the mystery of its effect was
at last explained.*
    —Sigmund Freud, *The Moses of Michelangelo*

There are more than two dozen references to madness in *Hamlet*, and
many more in Shakespeare's other plays. Yet, despite his superbly rich
language, Shakespeare uses a mere handful of terms to describe persons
for whose abnormal mental conditions we now have thousands. We
attribute this difference to scientific progress that now permits us to
understand that persons such as Hamlet or Lady Macbeth are, in fact,
literary examples of mentally ill persons displaying the symptoms of
schizophrenia and depression. In his introduction to the Pelican series
edition of *Hamlet*, Willard Farnham states: "Hamlet, indeed, may seem
to have been shaped to order for psychoanalysis."[1] But, surely, this is a
case of putting the cart before the horse, by all of three centuries.
"Twentieth-century psychologies," Farnham adds, "invite us to see
within Hamlet some severe seizure of the soul which is close to disease,
if not actually disease."[2] But the leap from a seizure of the soul to a
disease of the body is no less prodigious than the leap from religion to
science, from mental disease to brain disease.

I reject this modern, medicalized view of Hamlet's behavior. Instead,
I regard our psychiatric vocabulary as a type of pseudoscientific slang.
American English thus contains two classes of slang terms for mental
illness—one professional, the other popular; each of these classes contains hundreds of words, doing essentially the same work Shakespeare
accomplished with just a handful. Because our psychiatric-diagnostic
terms *conceal* human tragedies behind a veil of pseudomedical jargon,

and because our colloquial slang terms for lunacy *divert* us with imaginative metaphors, both *distract* us from the painful realities of the human condition. In contrast, by using language at once direct and allusive, unadorned yet rich, Shakespeare exhibits not only the method in, and the meaning of, madness, but also the motives of those who seek to define others as mad, thus illuminating the conflicts intrinsic to the human condition. To illustrate this thesis, I shall cite, with a minimum of commentary, some of Shakespeare's most powerfully moving psychiatric observations.[3]

Early in *Hamlet*, Polonius diagnoses Hamlet as mad:

Mad call I it, for, to define true madness,
What is't but to be nothing else but mad?
(2.2. 93-94)

Is Shakespeare telling us, at the very birth of the modern idea of insanity *as* illness, that there is no such thing as mental illness—that there is, in fact, nothing to define? I think so, for he has Polonius adding: "But let that go" (line 95).

Observe that when we describe a person as brave or cowardly, loyal or disloyal, we expect no additional definitions of conditions anterior to the behavior so classified that serve as its causes. A person behaves bravely because he is brave, not because braveness or some other condition causes him to do so. Shakespeare uses the word *mad* the same way we use the word *magnanimous*—that is, as an adjective to describe certain kinds of behaviors. What kinds? Actually, Shakespeare attaches the adjective *mad* to several behaviors, such as:

- Behaviors that seem strange to some persons, but not to others—for example, Othello's jealousy,

- Behaviors whose motives seem obscure, perhaps because they are deliberately concealed—for example, Hamlet's suspiciousness,

- Behaviors that appear to be bizarre or meaningless, perhaps because they hide a guilty secret—for example, Lady Macbeth's hallucinations,

- Behaviors that are the results of tragic miscalculation, leading to disappointment, frustration, and helplessness—for example, King Lear's depression,

- Behaviors that, though eccentric, endear the subject to, rather than alienate him from, those around him—for example, "the lunatic, the lover, and the poet, [who] are of imagination all compact",[4]

- Behaviors considered mad not (necessarily) because the person's conduct is abnormal, but because denominating him as insane serves the interests of the diagnostician—for example, Polonius's declaring that Hamlet is mad.

Two points need to be emphasized in this connection. First, that Shakespeare uses the word *mad* as part of ordinary language, much as he might use words such as *love*, *hate*, or *envy*. The other is that he alludes to the rich possibilities for deploying the term *madness* to obscure human motivation, deny moral agency, and dehumanize and destroy the person categorized as mad.

Although madness cannot be defined, the term *mad*, as Shakespeare demonstrates, is a useful linguistic device for conjuring up images of dangerous passions and devious motivations. Thus, as Hamlet is pondering the mystery of his father's sudden death and his mother's hasty remarriage, Horatio warns him that his preoccupation with the circumstances of his father's demise "might deprive your sovereignty of reason / And draw you into madness" (1.4. 73-74). But is Hamlet *drawn* into madness: that is, is madness something that happens to him? Or is he *defined* as mad: that is, is madness a medical-moral blemish others attribute to him? In Hamlet's case, perhaps a bit of both. As Hamlet begins to unravel his mother's and uncle's guilty secret, Polonius, eager to gain the culprits' favor, reassures them:

—that I have found
The very cause of Hamlet's lunacy.
(2.2.48-49)

Claudius is delighted:

O, speak of that! That do I long to hear.
(Line 50)

Claudius hastens to communicate the good news to Gertrude:

He [Polonius] tells me, my dear Gertrude, he hath found
The head and source of your son's distemper.
(Lines 54–55)

Then, with Polonius addressing Hamlet, Shakespeare pronounces these immortal words about madness as *motivated behavior*:

POLONIUS. Though this be madness, yet there is method
        in't.—Will you walk out of the air, my lord?
HAMLET. Into my grave?
POLONIUS. . . . How pregnant
        sometimes his replies are!
        (2.2. 203-7)

Realizing that his elders are trying to incriminate him as insane and hence irrational, Hamlet warns Guildenstern that two can play at that game as well as one—that irrationality may be a disguise and hence a form of calculated rationality.

HAMLET. I am but mad north-north-west. When the wind is
        southerly I know a hawk from a handsaw.
        (Lines 369-70)

Indeed, Claudius and Gertrude already suspect that Hamlet might be feigning madness to deceive them: They send for Hamlet's friends, Rosencrantz and Guildenstern, ostensibly to help him, but actually to discover his secret and to dispose of him.

THE KING [addressing Rosencrantz and Guildenstern].
And can you by no drift of conference
Get from him why he puts on this confusion,
Grating so harshly all his days of quiet
With turbulent and dangerous lunacy?
(3.1. 1-4)

GUILDENSTERN. Nor do we find him forward to be sounded,
But with crafty madness keeps aloof
When we would bring him on to some confession
Of his true state.
(Lines 5-9)

Meanwhile, Polonius escalates his psychiatric expertise: He now claims to have unraveled the etiology of Hamlet's madness as well:

But yet do I believe
The origin and commencement of his grief
Sprung from neglected love.
(Lines 176-79)

And he prescribes the cure: Remove, confine, and incapacitate the troublemaking madman.

POLONIUS [to the King]. To England send him, or confine him where
Your wisdom best shall think.

The King is duly alarmed:

It shall be so.
Madness in great ones must not unwatched go.
(Lines 188-89)

As act 3 draws to a close, Gertrude and Hamlet conduct the following remarkable colloquy.

GERTRUDE. This is the very coinage of your brain.
This bodily creation ecstasy . . .

HAMLET. Ecstasy?
My pulse as yours doth temperately keep time
. . . It is not madness
That I have uttered.
(3.4. 138-43)

Having let his mother know, or at least strongly suspect, that he has at last divined her guilty secret, Hamlet cautions her that he is anything but mad:

Make you to ravel all this matter out,
That I essentially am not in madness,
But mad in craft.
(Lines 187-89)

As Hamlet closes in on his quarries, Claudius and Gertrude grow more panicky and, once more, try to reassure themselves that Hamlet is mad. At the opening of act 4, Gertrude tells Claudius that Hamlet is,

Mad as the sea and wind when both contend. . . .
(Line 7)

Claudius agrees, but sees Hamlet as the avenger:

His liberty is full of threats to all,
To you yourself, to us, to every one.
(Lines 14-15)

Four lines later, Claudius calls Hamlet "This mad young man." Gertrude reciprocates with this telling metaphor:

> . . . his very madness, like some ore
> Among a mineral of metals base,
> Shows itself pure.
> (Lines 25-27)

In the meanwhile, Hamlet has killed Polonius, a deed Claudius quickly attributes to insanity:

> Hamlet in his madness hath Polonius slain.
> (Line 34)

It is difficult to imagine a person reading this play, or seeing it performed on the stage, interpreting Hamlet's stabbing Polonius as anything but a deliberate act and a dire warning to the Queen. The King is, indeed, planning a preemptive strike:

> How dangerous is it that this man goes loose!
> . . . Diseases desperate grown
> By desperate appliance are relieved,
> Or not at all.
> (4.3. 2-10)

Shakespeare's "desperate appliance" is an almost clairvoyant term for what we moderns regard as the scientific treatment of serious mental diseases, such as electroshock, lobotomy, and neuroleptic drugs.

The theme of madness, though it appears only toward the end of *Macbeth*, constitutes an extraordinarily powerful element of the tragedy. After Macbeth's successful climb to the pinnacle of political power, Lady Macbeth is overcome by guilt for her participation in her husband's murderous deeds. Her agitation and sleeplessness disturb Macbeth, who sends for a doctor to restore Lady Macbeth to what physicians would call her "premorbid condition." However, the doctor immediately recognizes that Lady Macbeth's hallucinations are the self-betrayals of her guilty secrets.

> DOCTOR [to Gentlewoman attendant]. Go to, go to! You have known what you should not.
> GENTLEWOMAN. She has spoke what she should not, I am sure of that.
> (5.1. 43-46)

The doctor, who has but a few lines in the play, consistently rejects Macbeth's effort to medicalize his wife's disturbance. "This disease," he insists, "is beyond my practice" (line 54). Then, he offers this explicit repudiation of the attempt to treat Lady Macbeth's disturbed behavior as a medical problem:

> Unnatural deeds
> Do breed unnatural troubles. Infected minds
> To their deaf pillows will discharge their secrets.
> More needs she the divine than the physician.
> God, God forgive us all! . . .
> I think, but dare not speak.
> (Lines 66-75)

When Macbeth enters the scene and demands that the doctor cure his wife, Shakespeare has the doctor say *exactly the opposite* of what—ever since the early 1800s, but especially since Freud's day—psychiatrists have been taught to think and say.

> MACBETH.How does your patient, doctor?
> DOCTOR. Not so sick, my lord,
> As she is troubled with thick-coming fancies
> That keep her from her rest.
> MACBETH.Cure her of that!
> Canst thou not minister to a mind diseased,
> Pluck from the memory a rooted sorrow,
> Raze out the written troubles of the brain,
> And with some sweet oblivious antidote
> Cleanse the stuffed bosom of that perilous stuff
> Which weighs upon her heart.
> DOCTOR. Therein the patient
> Must minister to himself.
> (5.8. 38-46)

2

The Contemporary Scene

Why is the concept of schizophrenia necessary at all? Firstly, because we have the term.
—World Health Organization

It has always seemed to me that the illnesses we call "mental" or "psychiatric" are analogies or similes. Accordingly, in *The Myth of Mental Illness*, I compared the difference between illness and mental illness to the difference between a genuine work of art and its imitation.[1] This distinction is simple enough, but there has been a remarkable resistance, in modern medicine, to applying the concepts of real and fake to diseases—though, revealingly, not to treatments.

When the valued object is a work of art or a scientific discovery, we accept the correlation between *originality* and *value* as a given, as something so obvious that it requires no further explanation.[2] However, when the thing valued is sickness (or the sick role), we behave as if something so generally dreaded as disease could never be an advantage. Nothing could be further from the truth. There are countless circumstances when being ill—or, better still, faking it—may benefit the subject. For example, illness (or the claim of being ill) may serve as an excuse (a white lie) for avoiding a social obligation; as a means of access to goods and services not available on the free market (prescription drugs, handicapped parking permits); as a source of sudden riches (a successful claim for compensation); or as a strategy for securing shelter and food (for the chronically mentally ill).

Why do people imitate works of art or fake behaviors? There are many reasons, the desire for financial gain usually being paramount. Once an object is deemed artistically (or scientifically) valuable, it is virtually certain to become economically valuable as well. In the modern world two important occurrences have made illness a valuable commodity, well worth faking. One is that the distinction between having an illness and

21

occupying the sick role has become increasingly blurred and, in our day, virtually nonexistent. The other is that being officially authenticated as sick—as a legitimate occupant of the sick role—has become increasingly useful and indeed often indispensable. Both of these developments began to gather momentum during the final decades of the nineteenth century and, in the United States, may now be reaching their apogee.

Indeed, that Freud's psychoanalytic language was analogic, through and through, was something both Karl Kraus and Ludwig Wittgenstein quickly recognized.[3] Sophie Freud, Sigmund Freud's granddaughter and professor of social work at Simmons College, has also emphasized this crucial characteristic of the language of psychoanalysis. Freud's metaphors, she wrote, "have seduced clinicians into treating mere ideas as facts or things."[4] The word *seduced* may be too generous here, as it excuses so-called clinicians (another misleading metaphor here) from their self-serving practice of transforming disapproved behaviors into disease entities. The result of this furious psychopathological entitification, to coin a term for it, dramatically illustrates Sir Walter Scott's famous admonition: "Oh, what a tangled web we weave,/ When first we practice to deceive!"[5]

The publication of Rudolf Virchow's *Cellular Pathology* in 1858 signaled the birth of medicine as a profession based on modern science. However, no sooner did the scientific criterion of illness become cellular pathology, than it began to be eroded by the claim that the "senseless" speech of mad persons was a "pathology of language," indicative of cellular pathology in the speaker's brain. Eugen Bleuler's invention of the idea of schizophrenia in 1911 completed the psychiatric transformation of language from a distinctively human characteristic into just another biological marker of brain disease.

In the eighteenth century, physicians only suspected that insanity was a genuine illness; today, they are sure of it. Yet, the evidence for this belief is still only the indisputable fact that most crazy people talk crazy. Thus, in a recent review of "the puzzle of schizophrenia," Julian Leff, a leading British psychiatrist, is forced to acknowledge that "the diagnostic concept remains fluid because there is no pathological test for schizophrenia."[6] For psychiatrists, it remains unthinkable that the crux of the matter may be not that there is no test for schizophrenia, but that there is no schizophrenia.[7] Leff concludes his essay with this important sentence:

"Nevertheless, there are still enough casualties of the system for anyone to form an opinion as to whether schizophrenia is a myth or a diagnostic entity by holding a *conversation* with their local bag lady or man."[8] In short, Leff rests his case on two glaring mistakes—confusing diagnoses with diseases and assuming that a conversation with a homeless person constitutes a valid scientific method for determining that the subject suffers from a brain disease.[9]

Of course, there have always been people who talked "crazy." Formerly, when our world view was theocentric, their behavior was viewed in religious terms and was called "the gift of tongues." Today, when our world view is medicocentric, such behavior is viewed in medical terms and is called a "symptom of schizophrenia" or "schizophrenese." J. R. Smythies, a prominent British psychiatrist, uses this criterion to diagnose James Joyce and Ludwig Wittgenstein as mentally/neurologically ill. He writes:

> Certain schizoid personalities develop the ability to write in a form of *speech disorder* known as schizophrenese. . . . A well-known example in literature is *Finnegan's Wake*. Joyce himself was never overtly schizophrenic . . . but he must have been near enough to it to be able to write schizophrenese (which normal people find almost impossible to do).[10]

After explaining that the essence of schizophrenic speech/writing disorder is that "the meaning of a statement is never quite contained within the statement," Smythies asserts "that Wittgenstein's philosophical writings exhibit [this characteristic] to a singular degree."[11] The leap from language to lesion implicit in this view is based only on faith, exactly as the leap from language to holiness, implicit in viewing glossolalia as "speaking in tongues," is based only on faith.

Actually, the phenomenon of people speaking in a seemingly unintelligible language has been observed in all ages and in all parts of the world.[12] In the Christian West, the practice, called "speaking in tongues," goes all the way back to the founding of this religion.[13] Today, it is especially common in the United States, mainly among Pentecostal Protestants, hundreds of thousands of whom occasionally engage in such behavior. Because such behavior expresses and evokes intense emotions, there is virtually no semantically neutral way of describing or defining it. Indeed, the various definitions of glossolalia illustrate how our language often frames and defines our "reality."

Webster's Third New International Dictionary defines glossolalia as: "ecstatic speech that is usually unintelligible to hearers and is uttered in worship services of various contemporary religious groups laying great stress on religious excitation and emotional fervor."[14] The *New Catholic Encyclopedia* offers: "A charisma that enables the recipient to praise God in miraculous speech."[15] According to the *Psychiatric Dictionary*, it is "tongue jabbering. Unintelligible jargon."[16] The authoritative *American Handbook of Psychiatry* states that it is the "mimicking [of] animal sounds or pronouncing meaningless neologisms" and is a common symptom of hysteria "occurring among Polar Eskimos."[17] Harold I. Kaplan and Benjamin J. Sadock, the editors of the standard American textbook of psychiatry, state that glossolalia is "the expression of a revelatory message through unintelligible words," and place it under the heading "Specific Disturbances in Forms of Thought," in a chapter titled "Typical Signs and Symptoms of Psychiatric Illness."[18] Finally, *The American Heritage Illustrated Encyclopedic Dictionary* defines glossolalia as "fabricated, incoherent, or nonsensical speech, especially as associated with certain schizophrenic syndromes."[19] In short, not just ordinary people but even authorities on language and medicine either canonize the phenomenon as holy, or demonize it as "a neurotic or psychotic symptom."[20]

However, we can reject these categorizations and view glossolalia anthropologically, as illustrative of one of the ways "man uses language when he practices religion."[21] Mutatis mutandis, the speech we execrate as "schizophrenese" is illustrative of how man uses language when he practices madness, and the speech we exalt as psychodiagnostics is illustrative of how man uses language when he practices psychiatry.

Classifying glossolalia and schizophrenese as nonsense *prejudges* the phenomena by defining them as nonmotivated actions—that is, as not behaviors but happenings, similar, say, to an epileptic seizure. But this is clearly false. The motives for religious and psychiatric glossolalia are obvious. Each is a semantic strategy for overcoming an actual or perceived social inferiority. The introductory verses of the First Letter of Paul to the Corinthians make this point clearly enough:

> For it is written, "I will destroy the wisdom of the wise, and the cleverness of the clever I will thwart." . . . God chose what is foolish in the world to shame the wise.[22]

In early Christianity, speaking in tongues was a manifestation of being "filled with the Holy Spirit"; today, in the Catholic Pentecostal movement, it is recognized as "of unassailable validity . . . of the fullness of life in the Spirit."[23] Similarly, in the nineteenth century, speaking in the tongue of psychodiagnostics proved that the speaker recognized madness as a medical malady; today, it is considered evidence of the validity of the view that mental illnesses are brain diseases.

The question remains: Why should we regard people who talk crazy as having a brain disease? Frustrated by what he regards as the success of my sustained argument showing that mental illnesses fail to meet the Virchowian criterion of disease, Sir Martin Roth complains: "Of course, if illness is a matter of lumps, lesions and germs most schizophrenics are perfectly healthy."[24] Indeed so. This is why psychiatrists need to add "pathological" language to pathological cells as markers indicative of the presence of illness. To be sure, people with strokes often exhibit impaired speech. But physicians do not use neurologically impaired speech (which differs in obvious ways from so-called psychotic speech) to establish that the diagnosis of stroke stands for a disease. They do that by finding the appropriate lesions in the brain at autopsy. It seems to me that no amount of reasoning or research can bridge the gap between tissue and talk, between cellular pathology and language pathology.

The proposition that a disorder of language is a disease of the brain is, prima facie, absurd. Language is a form of self-expression. There are many readily discernable reasons why there have always been, and always will be, persons who choose to express themselves in unconventional ways. Bleuler asserted that individuals denominated as insane talked crazy because they suffered from a brain disease. But if we regard speaking in unconventional ways as a symptom of a brain disease called "schizophrenia" (due to a "split" between thought and language), then we ought to regard painting in unconventional ways as a symptom of a brain disease called "schizovisia" (due to a "split" between seeing and representing).

I have remarked elsewhere on the historical reasons, conceptual confusions, and social context that lie at the heart of the idea of schizophrenia.[25] I return to this subject here because schizophrenia remains the paradigmatic metaphoric illness of modernity—a nonillness authoritatively declared to be a disease, generated and justified by our bafflement by what the Other qua Madman says (even when he does not address us). The upshot is that perhaps never before in history have so many educated people squandered so much effort on chasing after a pseudoscientific will-o-the-wisp as psychiatrists and psychologists have in studying "schizophrenia." In a comprehensive review of this awesome wasteland, Sherry Rochester and J. R. Martin note that there is something patently wrong with the initial assumptions on which the idea of schizophrenia rests. They write:

> In 1911, Eugen Bleuler reported his experience of being a confused listener in the presence of incoherent speakers. . . . To say that a speaker is incoherent is only to say that one cannot understand that speaker. So to make a statement about incoherent discourse is really to make a statement about one's own confusion as a listener.[26]

Undeterred by realizing that they have glimpsed the emperor's nakedness, the authors proceed to review a staggering number of studies, refusing to see that the point of this whole psychiatric enterprise is to legitimize schizophrenics as genuine patients, and the professionals who treat them as genuine healers:

> The study of the language use of schizophrenia has not been a happy enterprise. Every major reviewer in the last decade has observed that there is no adequate theory of why schizophrenic speakers produce aberrant discourse. . . . after some fifty years of effort, promising models and adequate data are still lacking in this field.[27]

But asking for a "theory of why schizophrenic speakers produce aberrant discourse" is like asking for a theory of why schizovisic painters (like Pablo Picasso or Jackson Pollock) produce aberrant pictures. People have *reasons* for what they do, not *theories* for producing what others deem "aberrant."

The error in the leap from aberrant self-expression to illness is obvious. Because the criterion of the modern, cellular concept of disease is a demonstrable bodily lesion, whether a person talks sense or nonsense is irrelevant for establishing whether he does or does not have a brain disease. If such a deviant style of self-expression were sufficient ground for establishing that the speaker has a brain disease, then deviant styles of other types of self-expression—such as dancing, music, and painting—would also have to be classified as the manifestations of brain disease. Nevertheless, the belief that a psychiatrist can examine a person's speech, as he can examine his spinal fluid, and can validly infer from it that the speaker's brain is diseased has become unquestioned medical dogma. Thus, as cardiologists recognize various disorders of the heart, so psychiatrists recognize various disorders of language—such as, Developmental Articulation Disorder, Elective Mutism, Phonological-Syntactic Disorder, Semantic-Pragmatic Deficit Disorder, and so forth.[28] I am not concerned here whether these terms correctly identify certain discrete speech patterns. For the sake of simplifying the argument, let us assume they do. I maintain, however, that the presence of speech patterns deemed to be psychopathological tells us no more about the brains of the persons who display such speech than the presence of various types of ordinary languages (such as English or German) tells us about the brains of persons who speak these languages.

Nevertheless, psychiatrists regard the view that schizophrenese is a language like a foreign tongue, rather than the manifestation of a disease like delirium, as patently false. Why? Because, in their view, schizophrenic language is, a priori, "gibberish," "meaningless," "word salad," in short, not understandable. To appreciate the crucial role of this premise it may be useful to compare language to light. Physicists distinguish between light by which we see (sodium light) and light that we see (neon light). Although the distinction is clear and useful, these categories are not mutually exclusive. The same is true for language. We can treat any person's speech as language or as nonlanguage—as meaningful communication containing clues about the speaker as moral agent or as meaningless noise containing clues about the speaker's brain disease. By assuming the latter stance toward speech classified as schizophrenic (or psychotic), psychiatrically diagnosed language disorders (like magnetic imaging techniques) become windows through which doctors can peer directly into the human brain—and discover what they always wanted to find: "Developmental language disorders . . . are the consequences of poorly understood static abnormalities of the immature brain. They have a number of etiologies, with genetics probably playing a more important role than perinatal insults."[29]

Thus, in modern biological psychiatry, it is no longer necessary to demonstrate the presence of a brain lesion in persons said to have a mental/brain disease. An authoritative diagnoses by psychiatrists of the speaker has replaced the need to find a cellular-pathological basis for the claimed disease.

The Eskimos have dozens of words for snow. The Chinese have more words for rice than for love. We have more words and phrases for mental illness than for any other idea, illness, or phenomenon. Despite this evidence of our own language, official medical and nonmedical authorities alike support the slogan that "mental illness is like any other illness," and ignore the ideological role of the idea of mental illness. For example, the authoritative five-volume *Dictionary of the History of Ideas* lists no entry for mental illness or any of its synonyms.[30] *Keywords: A Vocabulary of Culture and Society*, a work similar in scope though less extensive in size, also ignores mental illness and related terms.[31]

While English is an exceptionally rich language, most behaviors and things have only a few names. Bodily diseases usually have one or two medical names, as well as a few others in everyday language and perhaps slang. For mental diseases, however, we have thousands of words, some ostensibly scientific, others in ordinary language, still others in slang. This overabundance of terms for abnormal behaviors and our intemperate inclination to call people "sick" are symptoms of the thoroughgoing medicalization of life characteristic of contemporary American culture—a culture in which people give meaning to life by medicalizing it with psychiatric ideas, and manage interpersonal and social problems by means of mental health interventions.

Why is one of the most important *ideas* and *words* of our age not even mentioned in many encyclopedic and learned works on key ideas and key words? Anatole France might have answered by citing his celebrated caveat: "Les savants ne sont pas curieux." ("The savants are not curious"). I would add that the savants' curiosity falls below zero when open-mindedness threatens to lead them to conclusions they have rejected in advance. There is, indeed, good reason for the experts' a priori rejection of the proposition that mental illness exists only in the sense in which ghosts and witches exist.

Like a thick fog, professional mental health jargon prevents and protects us from seeing the futility of life and the limitations of the human condition. Our lexicon of medical metaphors for human misery and tragedy—with "mental illness" *primus inter pares*—conceals what, in bright light, is all too clearly visible. At the same time, by forcing us to strain to see better, these metaphors reveal features of the human landscape that might otherwise escape our attention. This dual function of slang merits some brief remarks.

Although all human beings speak a language, people in different countries typically speak different languages. Moreover, even people in the same country speak different versions of the same basic language, according to their occupation and social class. We call these various versions argot, cant, colloquialism, dialect, lingo, idiom, vernacular, euphemism, jargon, slang, and scientific or technical vocabulary. The boundaries separating slang or scientific language from everyday speech are loose and constantly shifting. Some slang terms—for example, *ghost writer*—are metaphors that capture the imagination and quickly make their way into everyday language; others—for example, *psychoanalysis*—satisfy our conceit that we are making progress in understanding something in the real world hitherto shrouded in mystery, when, in fact, we are merely coining a new word, and become a part of the language because they sound scientific.

What is the formal definition of *slang*? According to *Webster's Third New International Dictionary*, it is "language peculiar to a particular group . . . ; the special and often secret vocabulary used by a class . . . ; the jargon used by or associated with a particular trade, profession, or field of activity . . . extravagant, forced, or facetious figures of speech." I would add that, as Mencken emphasized, slang is also "a form of colloquial speech created in a spirit of defiance and aiming at freshness and novelty . . . [that] embodies a kind of social criticism."[32] Indeed, many slang expressions for mental illness—such as *bananas, a screw loose, not all there*—constitute a kind of counterlanguage, debunking untruths clothed in psychiatric jargon.

Preoccupation with mental health and ill health, reflected in contemporary American English, is a novel and peculiarly American phenomenon. While I am not as familiar with any other language as I am with American English, it is my impression, confirmed by persons at home in European languages, that no people have as rich a vocabulary for mental illness as we do. Also, there can be no doubt about the novelty of this phenomenon. Most of the slang words for mental illness in this lexicon are twentieth-century coinages. It is not hard to see why this should be so.

As human beings, we are, perforce, social creatures; which means that we must get along with one another, or suffer the consequences. Because we now live in a scientific age, we perceive our failures to get along with one another in scientific (or pseudoscientific) images, and articulate them in pseudomedical terms. Yet we cannot help but realize that our quintessentially human problems are utterly unlike the maladies into whose mold the language of mental health casts them. As a result, those who seek help in the psychiatric idiom become imprisoned by it, much as those who seek help in a mental hospital become imprisoned in it. Some people like, and ask, to be so constrained: The illusion of being able to understand and explain everyone's behavior—in a secret language that sets those who speak it apart from those who do not—makes the speakers feel secure and superior. Others chafe at the restraints: Feeling imprisoned in a semantic straitjacket, they oppose their keepers and make their escape by generating a rich vocabulary of slang for mental illnesses.

A fingerprint, unlike a photograph, identifies a person uniquely. The same is true for a culture's—or subculture's or profession's—vocabulary: No two of them use the same words the same way. Americans and Australians, diplomats and doctors, criminals and lawyers, chemists and computer programmers all have their specialized lexicons. Some jargon terms are understood by competent speakers of the root language; others, only by insiders. For example, when a physician says he is *palpating* a woman's breast for the presence of a tumor, a lay person knows that the doctor is *touching and feeling* her breast, but is using a euphemism to say so. But when a psychiatrist declares that an old woman in a nursing home has a *bipolar illness,* or that a young man who has dropped out of college has *schizophrenia*, a lay person thinks the doctor has made a diagnosis and does not realize that, in fact, he has merely renamed these persons. People thus do not realize that the old woman is unhinged because death is all she has left to live for; and that the young man is unhinged because he has a long life ahead of him, but has not the faintest idea what to do with it.

Psychiatrists spend many years learning their specialized language whose authoritative use distinguishes them from other physicians and lay persons. Under the heavy weight of habit and self-interest, they are likely to be taken in by their own jargon and believe that persons called "mental patients" *have* brain diseases, that *cause* them to have mental diseases. The possibility that mental diseases are merely names no longer occurs to them or to other normally socialized people.

Still, most of the time people know perfectly well what constitutes a real disease—for example, lung cancer or myocardial infarction. Regardless of what a person may call himself, or what others may call him, if he has lung cancer or a heart attack, the chances are that the disease will kill him. This is not true for mental illnesses. For example, depression cannot kill a person. Of course, a person can always kill himself, and psychiatrists can always attribute his suicide to depression. Similarly, schizophrenia cannot make a person shoot a president or cause him to be incarcerated in a mental hospital. But, again, a person can always decide to shoot, or try to shoot, the president; and psychiatrists can always attribute his act to insanity, incarcerate him, and call his confinement "hospitalization." Everyone knows this. And hardly anyone gives the matter serious second thoughts. Why? Because whether we treat a wrenching human predicament as an existential problem or as a medical problem entails a choice that we like to pretend is not a choice. Here is a classic example.

A young woman delivers her first baby, a beautiful, healthy infant. The next morning she weeps, has no appetite, says she is unhappy, and displays a mood of dejection. What do we say about her? Is she ill? Clearly, we have a wide range of words, phrases, and figures of speech from which to choose to describe the distraught mood and behavior of such a person. We could say that she is sad, unhappy, angry, melancholy, blue, depressed, desperate, or suicidal; or that she does not want to grow up, rejects the baby, fears motherhood, or avoids confronting the conflict between career and family; or that she is ill, suffering from postpartum depression, postpartum psychosis, acute schizophrenia, or toxic-organic psychosis due to endocrine imbalance; and so forth. Each of these terms and phrases identifies the same phenomenon; each word and phrase is at once a *name* and an *explanation*. We can thus ask: Which explanation is true? Or: Why do we have a vocabulary that identifies a woman who is happy with her newborn baby as *healthy*, and one who is unhappy with it as *sick*?

It is clear that most educated persons recognize that bodily diseases are biological defects or malfunctions of the body; in short, that they are facts, in the same sense that defects or malfunctions of a dog's body are diseases and facts.

It is not clear, however, what people think mental diseases are. Do they think mental illnesses are the same as physical diseases, that is, diseases of the brain? Or that they are some other kinds of diseases? Or that they are not really diseases at all?

It seems to me that many people—physicians and lay persons, educated and uneducated persons alike—are of two minds about mental
illnesses and everything connected with them: They believe that mental
illnesses are and are not real diseases; that psychiatrists are and are not
real doctors;[33] that there is and is not any difference between psychiatrists
and clinical psychologists; that psychotherapy is "just talking" and
genuine therapy; that alcoholism is a bad habit and a genetically caused
disease; that psychiatric institutions are hospitals and prisons; that persons who commit criminal acts and are acquitted on the grounds of
insanity are bad and mad, guilty and innocent.

To be sure, most people tacitly understand that the psychiatrist's job
is to control deviance but pretend that he treats disease, to manage
misbehavior but make believe that he cures disease. However, the
institutionalized pretense perplexes, leaving people curious, confused,
and uneasy about mental illness. Thus, even educated and intelligent
people fear losing their minds, as if one's mind were like one's wallet
that one could mislay, and perhaps recover. Others believe that an
individual can have multiple personalities, as if personality were like a
letter that could be xeroxed, and thus one could have one or more copies
of it.

Having many words for mental illness is both a cause and a consequence of this confusion. Giving a problem in living a medical name is
a very mixed blessing. Calling (mis)behavior "illness" implies that a
doctor might be able to treat, if not cure, the malady, and is therefore
reassuring. On the other hand, wrapping human problems in medical
metaphors inhibits people from assuming responsibility for managing
their own lives, and is therefore disempowering and anxiety-producing.
In fact, so profound is the popular confusion about mental illness that
people no longer realize that the word *mind*, as a noun, is itself a
metaphor. We have a liver, a heart, a spleen, and a brain—but we have
no mind. Only as a verb does the word *mind* have a literal meaning, as
in phrases such as "who is *minding* the store?" or "*mind* your own
business!"

How do we know that a person *has* a mental illness? I use this awkward
phrasing because the introduction to the third edition of the American
Psychiatric Association's *Diagnostic and Statistical Manual of Mental
Disorders* (*DSM-III*) specifically states: "A common misconception is
that a classification of mental disorders classifies individuals, when

actually what are being classified are disorders that *individuals have*."[34] Evidently, the official American manufacturers of mental disorders are so fond of this phrase that they reprinted it verbatim in *DSM-III-R*.[35]

Of course, there is no blood or other biological test to ascertain the presence or absence of a mental illness, as there is for most bodily diseases. If such a test were developed (for what, theretofore, had been considered a psychiatric illness), then, as I noted earlier, the condition would cease to be a mental illness and would be classified, instead, as a symptom of a bodily disease.

How, then, do we know that a particular person has a mental illness? We know it the same way we know that a painting "has" beauty or value: Because someone in authority says so, and because we believe him. This difference between the way we *determine a fact* and *define an attribution* explains why no educated person would say "I know diabetes when I see it," but educated persons do not hesitate to say, and say with conviction, "I know obscenity when I see it," or "I know schizophrenia when I see it." The difficulty with this method of "knowing" by "seeing" is that what a person sees depends in large part on who he is. A lay person looking at an x-ray film sees only lights and shadows; whereas a radiologist looking at it may see cancer or pneumonia. Neil Postman offers the following example to illustrate the problem. Three baseball umpires compare notes:

> The first umpire, being a man of small knowledge of how meanings are made, says, "I calls 'em as they are." The second umpire, knowing something about human perception and its limitations, says, "I calls 'em as I sees 'em." The third umpire, having studied at Cambridge with Wittgenstein himself, says, "Until I calls 'em, they ain't."[36]

Fortunately, we can do something more: We can observe the game—whether baseball or life itself—and pit our own knowledge and common sense against the pronouncements of the experts, the politicians, and "what everyone knows." The ever-present availability of this countervailing force is nicely captured in a parable attributed to Abraham Lincoln: "If you call a tail a leg, how many legs has a dog?" "Five." "No, four, because calling a tail a leg doesn't make it a leg."

The value of the story about the baseball umpires thus lies in alerting us to the role of authority and power in naming: "Until I calls 'em, they ain't." Thus, a patient may cancel his appointment with a psychoanalyst because of a pressing obligation, but the analyst may "interpret"—that is, attribute —this act as being motivated by the patient's fear of discovering more about himself. Similarly, a person may be saddened because of his unhappiness with his wife, but a psychiatrist may "diagnose"—that is attribute—his mood as being caused by a clinical depression requiring drug treatment. The thing we must remember is that, although no one *is* anything until someone so identifies him, this fact (inherent in our being language-using moral agents) does not, ipso facto, tell us whether he is what he has been called or something else. We can have differences of opinion about social attributions, and even about so-called facts. However, a "false fact" is not a fact at all; it is an error. The difference between diagnosing a person as *having* hysteria and as *having* malaria is therefore similar to the difference between having an opinion and affirming a fact. The comic effect of an old and once-famous joke about the psychoanalyst's diagnoses of his patients derives from this source: If the patient is early, he is anxious; if he is late, he is hostile; and if he is on time, he is compulsive. Opinion is all-important. Truth is irrelevant.

This form of authoritative opinionatedness, often bordering on the absurd, has a long history. In the past, the persons rendering pompous opinions were typically priests: Intoxicated with God, they attributed divine causation to every event in the universe. Today, the opinionated persons are likely to be biological psychiatrists: Intoxicated with (pseudo)science, they attribute scientific causation to all human events—which, for so-called mental events, means psychopathological causation. Freud's *Psychopathology of Everyday Life* is a classic example of this posture.[37]

James Strachey, the editor of Freud's collected works, correctly emphasized that Freud intended this work as proof of "the universal application of determinism to mental events,"[38] in other words, proof that psychoanalysis is a bona fide science of the mind. This view complemented and supported the then burgeoning psychiatric view that every behavioral pattern that psychiatrists identify ("diagnose") as a mental disease is, in fact, a manifestation of a brain disease. This effort to medicalize life is every bit as erroneous, and ridiculous, as the effort to theologize life, for which it is a pseudoscientific substitute.[39]

To be sure, science plays a crucial role in providing the infrastructure of our *physical* existence. But it plays a very subordinate role—and this may surprise many educated people today—in forming the structure of our *social* existence. Love and hate, loyalty and betrayal, intemperance and self-discipline, productivity and parasitism—these and our other personal *dispositions* and *qualities* have little or nothing to do with science. So much the worse for science. However, the fact that something in the world is not subject to scientific analysis or control does not mean that we cannot look at it carefully and describe it truthfully. Honesty is not a scientific concept, yet it is the slender reed on which science itself rests.

In recent decades, it has become more fashionable than ever for psychiatrists to declare, ostensibly on the basis of new "evidence," that one or another mental disease is not really a disease; and also to insist that some pattern of behavior, hitherto not identified as a disease, is in fact a mental disease. These pronouncements, published in scientific journals, are accepted as if they were discoveries; and they are ballyhooed by the press as if they were medical breakthroughs. For example, some twenty years ago, the membership of the American Psychiatric Association, discovered, by a relatively narrow *vote*, that homosexuality is not a disease. More recently, some experts have discovered that alcoholism is also not a disease. However, the majority of the discoveries concerning mental diseases go the other way—for example, affirming that adultery is a disease (sex addiction), or that smoking is a disease (tobacco dependence).

However, such claims are not based on empirical observations, should not be confused with discoveries, and are simply decisions about how to use words such as *disease* and *treatment*.[40] To put it differently, real doctors (for example, pathologists) *discover* real diseases (for example, AIDS) by working on the human body; whereas fake doctors (psychiatrists) *coin* metaphoric diseases (for example, tobacco dependence), by working on a society's vocabulary. I categorize the second group of maladies as metaphoric rather than literal diseases. But are they such? Who decides whether language is used literally or metaphorically? Is schizophrenia a metaphor? Is God? Did He literally give Moses the Ten Commandments, or is that merely a figure of speech?

Nowadays, most of us, most of the time, have little trouble dealing with such examples, provided they are drawn from the vocabulary of religion and theology. Usually, we think about such things one way as children, and another way as adults, by which time we have learned that, while we can think what we please about religion, we should say nothing about it, or only what others want to hear. Correct social behavior requires that we let sleeping religious metaphors lie. What happens when they are awakened and become active in the world?

We know only too well what happens when religious metaphors are aroused, as recent events in Iran, Iraq, Israel, and Lebanon illustrate. Metaphors are literalized, words turn into weapons, their users acquire armaments, and the rest is history—mayhem and murder, in the name of God. Replace God with mental illness, the favorite metaphor of modern people, and observe a similar process at work.

The pattern is set in childhood, exemplified by the following typical dialogue. A young boy, playing with a toy horse, says to his mother: "Look at my horsie." His mother replies: "Oh, that is a nice horse. What is his *name*?" Child and adult both know that the toy is not a horse. But their reciprocally validated pretense creates a kind of reality. *Mutatis mutandis*, a woman—perhaps a "child" in the body of an adult, to coin another metaphor—"toys" with her life. She tells her social worker that she has seven personalities, one of whom was raped the night before by her boyfriend. Psychiatrists, judges, and the press eagerly validate the woman's pretense. They tell her the *name* of her illness. And we are off to a deadly game of literalized medical metaphors. Once again, the words become weapons—ostensibly against diseases, but actually against persons. Their users acquire a real therapeutic "armamentarium"—chemicals, convulsions, confinements, and coercions called "treatments." And the medicalized meddlers, fortified with their politically legitimized slang, go out into the world to do good—in the name of Mental Health. To me, the whole affair looks like more mayhem and murder.

In my opinion, the entire vocabulary of psychiatry is pseudoscientific slang. The difference between the scientific-sounding terms of *DSM-III-R*, journalistic psychobabble, and outright slang is wholly a matter of *legitimacy*. Scientific journals and prestigious newspapers, doctors and insurance companies, lawyers and the United States Supreme Court all recognize official psychiatric language as medical and scientific; whereas any idiom labeled "jargon" or "psychobabble" is, ipso facto, not scientific. To be sure, a good slang term may convey more truth than its pseudoscientific synonym. But truth, as I noted earlier, has nothing to do with the matter.

3

Dictionaries of Deviance

*He's mad that trusts in the tameness of a wolf, a
horse's health, a boy's love, or a whore's oath.*
—Shakespeare, *King Lear*

DSM-III-R: The Official Roster of Mental Disorders

*Mental health problems do not affect three or
four out of every five persons, but one out of one.*
—William Menninger, *New York Times*

*[A]ll people have mental illness of different de-
grees at different times, and sometimes some are
much worse, or better.*
—Karl Menninger, *The Vital Balance*

In 1980, the American Psychiatric Association (APA) published the
third edition of its *Diagnostic and Statistical Manual of Mental Disorders*
(*DSM-III*).[1] This document was celebrated for its deletion of homosexuality from the list of mental disorders, and was hailed as the symbol of
the new, "medical" psychiatry. Yet, only three years later—ostensibly
because "data were emerging from new studies that were inconsistent
with some of the diagnostic criteria"—the APA embarked on a revision
of *DSM-III*, which was published in 1987.[2] A year later, the Board of
Trustees of the APA appointed a Task Force to prepare DSM-IV. In 1991,
the APA published *DSM-IV Options Books: Work in Progress.*[3] DSM-IV
is scheduled for publication in 1994. More than ever, the profession of
psychiatry seems determined to ground its medical legitimacy on creating diagnoses and pretending that they are diseases.

The APA's *furor diagnosticus* has led even some mainstream psychiatrists to question the association's motives for publishing one version
of the *DSM* after another. A poll of the membership of the APA soliciting

its opinion about the frequent revisions of its diagnoses revealed that "20% of a random sample of American psychiatrists believed that income for the APA was a major reason for publishing *DSM-III-R*."[4] P. T. Barnum is alleged to have said: "A sucker is born every minute." And a person to suckerize him, I might add, is born every second. I believe the APA's motives for manufacturing diagnoses are mainly existential and professional—that is, the desire to prove that psychiatrists are not quacks (pretending to be bona fide physicians), but real doctors (whose patients have real diseases). However, in health care, existential and economic concerns, like Siamese twins, are inseparable. My point is that real doctors do not have to go looking for diseases. The diseases—or, rather, the patients suffering and dying from them—find them soon enough. This is not true in psychiatry. Thus, before homosexuals were struck down by AIDS as a disease, they were struck down by homosexuality as a diagnosis. Ironically, now that AIDS is killing tens of thousands of persons, among them a disproportionate number of homosexuals, psychiatrists, in an arrogant attempt to rewrite history, insist that homosexuality is not a disease. My point is that virtually all psychiatric diagnoses are economic and political *claims*, serving the interests of psychiatry as a state-protected monopoly for the manufacture of pseudomedical euphemisms and dysphemisms. Understanding the meaning and function of such uplifting and downcasting terms is thus essential for understanding the meaning and function of psychiatric diagnoses.

Webster's defines *euphemism* as "The substitution of an inoffensive or mild expression for one that may offend or suggest something unpleasant. . . . as 'passing away' for 'dying.'" A *dysphemism*—which *Webster's* does not list and may be my own creation—is the opposite of a euphemism: for example, calling abortion "murder." Psychiatric jargon is a melange of euphemisms and dysphemisms, mainly the latter. Moreover, an expression may be regarded as a euphemism at one time, and as a dysphemism at another time. Psychiatrists are not alone in using words as instruments of legitimation and illegitimation. At this very moment, the people in the former Soviet Union and Eastern Europe are engaged in a similar enterprise—for example, renaming Leningrad as St. Petersburg.

Unlike regular physicians, who have no need to rename diabetes or hypertension, psychiatrists labor under the unremitting pressure of cultural forces to slap approving or disapproving labels on certain behaviors.

With women's liberation, nymphomania, formerly a "sexual perversion," has become normal behavior; whereas smoking, formerly *de rigueur* among psychiatrists, is now a disreputable mental disorder called "tobacco dependence." As nearly everyone realizes, much of the current preoccupation with "political correctness" centers on the use of language. In the resulting word games, some persons and acts are prettified, others uglified. Cripples become the handicapped, the disabled, and the differently abled. Lechery becomes sexual harassment, seduction is redefined as rape. Similarly, Negroes become blacks, and blacks, African-Americans. Each new term starts out life as a euphemism, and expires as a dysphemism. Hardly a day passes that the media do not report the new, semantically correct, terminology. As I write this, a report in the *New York Times* informs us that retarded persons—estimated to number 7.5 million Americans—are rejecting the term *retarded*: "Frustrated by what it considers the stigma of the word 'retarded,' delegates to a convention of the Association for Retarded Citizens of the United States voted to change the group's name to 'The Arc.'" Jim Gardner, president of the group, asked rhetorically: "We quit using 'idiot' and 'imbeciles,' so why do we have to use 'retarded?'"[5] This example strikes me as particularly instructive, showing that even retarded persons are shrewd enough to realize that although words, unlike sticks and stones, cannot break their bones—they can destroy them as persons. If nonretarded Americans fail to realize this, it is not because they are stupid, but because they collude with the members of the Hindering Professions in worshipping Mental Health—and wage war with psychiatric words.

DSM-III-R Classification of Mental Disorders[6]

Disorders usually first evident in infancy, childhood, or adolescence

Developmental Disorders

Mild mental retardation
Moderate mental retardation
Severe mental retardation
Profound mental retardation
Unspecified Mental Retardation

Pervasive Developmental Disorders

Autistic disorder
Pervasive developmental disorder
  not otherwise specified [NOS]

*Specific Developmental
Disorders*

Developmental arithmetic disorder
Developmental expressive writing
  disorder
Developmental reading disorder
Developmental articulation disorder
Developmental expressive language
  disorder
Developmental receptive language
  disorder
Developmental coordination disorder
Specific developmental disorder NOS

Disruptive Behavior Disorders

Attention-deficit hyperactivity disorder (ADHD)

Conduct Disorder

Solitary aggressive type
Undifferentiated type
Oppositional defiant disorder

*Anxiety Disorders of Childhood or
Adolescence*

Separation anxiety disorder
Avoidant disorder of childhood or ad-
  olescence
Overanxious disorder

*Other Disorders of Infancy, Child-
hood, or Adolescence*

Reactive attachment disorder of in-
  fancy
Schizoid disorder of childhood or ad-
  olescence
Elective mutism
Oppositional disorder
Identity disorder

Eating Disorders

Anorexia nervosa
Bulimia nervosa
Pica
Rumination disorder of infancy
Eating disorder NOS

Gender identity disorders

Gender identity disorder of childhood
Transsexualism
Gender identity disorder of adoles-
  cence or adulthood, non-
  transsexual type (GIDAANT)
Gender identity disorder NOS

Tic disorders

Tourette's disorder
Chronic motor or vocal tic disorder

Transient tic disorder
Tic disorder NOS

Elimination Disorders

Functional encopresis
Functional enuresis

Speech disorders not elsewhere classified

Cluttering
Stuttering

Other disorders of infancy, childhood, or adolescence

Elective mutism
Identity disorder
Reactive attachment disorder of infancy or early childhood
Stereotypy / Habit disorder
Undifferentiated attention-deficit disorder

Organic mental syndromes and disorders

Primary Degenerative Dementia of the Alzheimer Type, Senile Onset
　With delirium
　With delusion
　With depression
　Uncomplicated
Multi-infarct Dementia
　With delirium
　With delusion
　With depression
　Uncomplicated
Senile dementia NOS
Presenile dementia NOS

Psychoactive substance-induced organic mental disorders

Alcohol intoxication
Alcohol idiosyncratic intoxication
Uncomplicated alcohol withdrawal
Alcohol withdrawal delirium
Alcohol hallucinosis
Alcohol amnestic disorder
Dementia associated with alcoholism
Amphetamine or similarly acting sympathomimetic intoxication
Amphetamine or similarly acting sympathomimetic withdrawal
Amphetamine or similarly acting sympathomimetic delirium
Amphetamine or similarly acting sympathomimetic delusional disorder
Caffeine intoxication
Cannabis intoxication
Cannabis delusional disorder
Cocaine intoxication
Cocaine withdrawal
Cocaine delirium
Cocaine delusional disorder
Hallucinogen hallucinosis
Hallucinogen delusional disorder
Hallucinogen mood disorder
Posthallucinogen perception disorder
Inhalant intoxication[7]
Nicotine withdrawal
Opioid intoxication
Opioid withdrawal
Phencyclidine (PCP) or similarly acting arylcyclohexylamine intoxication
Phencyclidine (PCP) or similarly acting arylcyclohexylamine delirium

Phencyclidine (PCP) or similarly acting arylcyclohexylamine delusional disorder

Phencyclidine (PCP) or similarly acting arylcyclohexylamine mood disorder

Phencyclidine (PCP) or similarly acting arylcyclohexylamine organic mental disorder NOS

Sedative, hypnotic, or anxiolytic intoxication

Uncomplicated sedative, hypnotic, or anxiolytic withdrawal

Sedative, hypnotic, or anxiolytic withdrawal delirium

Sedative, hypnotic, or anxiolytic amnestic disorder

Other unspecified psychoactive substance intoxication

Other unspecified psychoactive substance withdrawal

Other unspecified psychoactive substance delirium

Other unspecified psychoactive substance dementia

Other unspecified psychoactive substance amnestic disorder

Other unspecified psychoactive substance delusional disorder

Other unspecified psychoactive substance hallucinosis

Other unspecified psychoactive substance mood disorder

Other unspecified psychoactive substance anxiety disorder

Other unspecified psychoactive substance personality disorder

Other unspecified psychoactive substance organic mental disorder NOS

Organic Mental Disorders Associated with Axis III Physical Disorders or Conditions, Whose Etiology Is Unknown

Delirium

Dementia

Amnestic disorder

Organic delusional disorder

Organic hallucinosis

Organic mood disorder

Organic anxiety disorder

Organic personality disorder

Organic mental disorder NOS

Psychoactive substance use disorders

Alcohol dependence

Alcohol abuse

Amphetamine or similarly acting sympathomimetic dependence

Amphetamine or similarly acting sympathomimetic abuse

Cannabis dependence

Cannabis abuse

Hallucinogen dependence

Hallucinogen abuse

Inhalant dependence

Inhalant abuse

Nicotine dependence

Opioid dependence

Opioid abuse

Phencyclidine (PCP) or similarly acting arylcyclohexylamine dependence

Phencyclidine (PCP) or similarly acting arylcyclohexylamine abuse

Sedative, hypnotic, or anxiolytic dependence

Sedative, hypnotic, or anxiolytic abuse

Polysubstance dependence

Polysubstance dependence NOS

Polysubstance abuse NOS

Schizophrenia

Catatonic type

Disorganized type

Paranoid type

Undifferentiated type

Residual type

Delusional (Paranoid) Disorder

Psychotic disorders not elsewhere classified

Brief reactive psychosis

Schizophreniform disorder

Schizoaffective disorder

Induced psychotic disorder

Psychotic disorder NOS (Atypical psychosis)

Mood disorders

Bipolar disorder, mixed

Bipolar disorder, manic

Bipolar disorder, depressed

Cyclothymia

Bipolar disorder NOS

Depressive Disorders

Major depression, single episode

Major depression, recurrent

Dysthymia (or Depressive neurosis)

Depressive disorder NOS

Anxiety disorders (or anxiety and phobic neuroses)

Panic disorder with agoraphobia

Panic disorder without agoraphobia

Agoraphobia without history of panic disorder

Social phobia

Simple phobia

Obsessive compulsive disorder (or Obsessive compulsive neurosis)

Posttraumatic stress disorder

Generalized anxiety disorder

Anxiety disorder NOS

Somatoform disorders

Body dysmorphic disorder (dysmorphobia)

Conversion disorder (or Hysterical neurosis, conversion type)

Hypochondriasis (or Hypochondriacal neurosis)

Somatization disorder

Somatoform pain disorder

Undifferentiated somatoform disorder

Somatoform disorder NOS

Dissociative disorders (or hysterical neuroses, dissociative type)

Multiple personality disorder

Psychogenic fugue

Psychogenic amnesia

Depersonalization disorder (or Depersonalization neurosis)

Dissociative disorder NOS

Sexual disorders

Exhibitionism

Fetishism

Frotteurism

Pedophilia
Sexual masochism
Sexual sadism
Transvestic fetishism
Paraphilia NOS

Sexual Dysfunctions

Hypoactive sexual desire disorder
Sexual aversion disorder
Female sexual arousal disorder
Male erectile disorder
Inhibited female orgasm
Inhibited male orgasm
Premature ejaculation
Dyspareunia
Vaginismus
Atypical psychosexual dysfunction
Sexual dysfunction NOS
Sexual disorder NOS

Sleep disorders

Insomnia related to another mental
    disorder (Nonorganic)
Insomnia related to a known organic
    factor
Primary insomnia
Hypersomnia related to another men-
    tal disorder (Nonorganic)
Hypersomnia related to a known or-
    ganic factor
Primary hypersomnia
Sleep-wake schedule disorder
Dyssomnia NOS
Dream anxiety disorder (Nightmare
    disorder)
Sleep terror disorder
Sleepwalking disorder
Parasomnia NOS

Factitious disorders

Factitious disorder with psychologi-
    cal symptoms
Factitious disorder NOS

Impulse control disorders not else-
where classified

Intermittent explosive disorder
Kleptomania
Pathological gambling
Pyromania
Trichotillomania
Impulse control disorder NOS

Adjustment disorder

Adjustment disorder with anxious
    mood
Adjustment disorder with depressed
    mood
Adjustment disorder with distur-
    bance of conduct
Adjustment disorder with mixed dis-
    turbance of emotions and conduct
Adjustment disorder with mixed emo-
    tional features
Adjustment disorder with physical
    complaints
Adjustment disorder with withdrawal
Adjustment disorder with work (or
    academic) inhibition
Adjustment disorder NOS

Psychological factors affecting
physical condition

Psychological factors affecting physi-
    cal condition

Personality disorders

Paranoid personality disorder
Schizoid personality disorder

Schizotypal personality disorder
Antisocial personality disorder
Borderline personality disorder
Histrionic personality disorder
Narcissistic personality disorder
Avoidant personality disorder
Dependent personality disorder

Obsessive compulsive personality disorder
Passive aggressive personality disorder
Personality disorder NOS

Codes for Conditions Not Attributable to a Mental Disorder That Are a Focus of Attention or Treatment

Academic problem
Adult antisocial behavior
Borderline intellectual functioning
Childhood or adolescent antisocial behavior
Malingering
Marital problem
Noncompliance with medical treatment

Occupational problem
Parent-child problem
Other interpersonal problem
Other specified family circumstances
Phase of life problem or other life circumstance problem
Uncomplicated bereavement

Additional Codes

Unspecified mental disorder (non-psychotic)
No diagnosis or condition on Axis I

Diagnosis or condition deferred on Axis I
No diagnosis on Axis II
Diagnosis deferred on Axis II

Synonyms for Mental Illness

> *So blind was the world, that, under whatever*
> *name the vain toys were presented, they were at*
> *once received without examination and selection*
> *as genuine. In this way, men made no difficulty in*
> *hugging any ass's or dog's bones which any*
> *trifler chose to bring forward, as the bones of*
> *martyrs.*
>
> —John Calvin,
> "Advantages from an
> Inventory of Relics"

The various terms listed in this catalogue mirror the fact that English-speaking people have long ago fallen into the habit of labeling as "crazy" virtually every kind of unusual or distasteful behavior, as well as anyone who displays such behavior. The result is an amazingly richly nuanced vocabulary for identifying, belittling, jeering, mocking, scorning, denigrating, and otherwise belittling and dismissing aberrant acts and deviant persons. Some of these terms have an amiable, indulgent feel to them—for example, *bent out of shape* or *flipped out*. Others are cruel and demeaning—for example, *berserk* or *sexual psychopath*. Such terms defy lexical definitions. The test of understanding them lies in intuitively grasping their conventional use, and in instinctively knowing, should one be so inclined, how to use them effectively.

A

Abalienation
Aberrance, Aberrancy
Aberration
Abnormal
Abnormalism
Abuse
    Alcohol abuse[8]
    Drug abuse
    Child abuse
    Elder abuse
    Granny abuse
    Psychotropic drug abuse
    Self-abuse
    Sex abuse

    Spouse abuse
    Substance abuse
    Wife abuse
Acid head
Acromania
Actual neurosis
Addiction (addict; *see also* -oholic)[9]
Addlebrained
Addled egg
Addledhead
Addlepated
Adventurism
Affective disorder
Agitation
Agoraphobia[10]
Ahasuerus's syndrome

Airhead

Alarmism

Alcohol abuse. *See also* separate list for Drunkenness, beginning on page 81

Alcohol dependence

Alcoholism

Algolagnia (sexual pleasure in suffering or inflicting physical pain; sadomasochism)

Alienation

All in his head

All worked up

Amentia

Amenty

Amnesia

Amphierotism (bisexualism)

An elephant in the moon

Anecdotage

Anhedonia

Anility, e.g., of old woman

Animal (e.g., he is an animal)

Anorexia

Anorexia nervosa

Anorgasmia

Anxiety neurosis

Apartment to let

Ape

Ape-shit

Aphrodisia

Apish

Apple sauce (full of)

Around the bend (e.g., he's gone around the bend)

Artifactual illness

Asberger's syndrome (collecting "meaningless" objects)

Asinine

Ass

Ass hole

Asthenia

At his wit's end

Athedonia (anhedonia, inability to be happy)

Atrabilarian (a sad and gloomy individual)

Attention deficit disorder (Hyperactivity)

Atypical

Authoritarian personality

Authoritarianism

Autism

Autoeroticism

Autolatry (the worship of oneself)

Automatism

Autophoby

Autotheism (a person's elevation of himself into being his own God; grandiosity; megalomania)

B

Babbler

Babbling

Babyhood

Bag of nuts

Bakehead

Balloonatic

Balminess

Balmy

Balmy in the crumpet

Bananas

Barbiturism

Balmy

Balmy on the crumpet

Basket case

Bean

Bet

Bats (e.g., he's got bats in the belfry)

Batted

Battered wife syndrome

Battering

Batty

Be derailed

Beans are in flower
Beany
Bedbug
Bedeviled
Bedlamism
Bedlamite
Bee in his bonnet (e.g., he has a . . .)
Bee in his head
Been working too hard
Beezy-weezies
Being a bug
Being on the bug
Belongs in a zoo
Benighted
Bent
Bent all out of shape
Bent out of shape
Bereft of reason
Berserk
Beside oneself
Bestiality
Bewilderment
Bewitched
Biddy (e.g., old biddy; used dis-
    paragingly, especially in reference
    to old women)
Bilge
Bipolar illness
Bird (e.g., he is a strange bird)
Bird seed
Bisexualism
Black dog on [one's] back
Blasted blind bat
Block
Block head
Blogo
Blooming idiot
Blow a fuse
Blow a gasket
Blow off steam
Blow one's cork
Blow one's lid

Blow one's lump
Blow one's stack
Blow one's top
Blow one's topper
Blue (e.g., in a blue funk; got the
    blues)
Blue funk
Blue Monday
Blunt-witted
Boggled (e.g., his mind is boggled)
Bogyism
Bolts-and-nuts
Bombed
Bombed out
Bonehead
Bongo
Bonkers
Booby
Booze-wacky
Borderline (e.g., personality)
Bovine
Bovinity
Bozo
Brainless
Brains are fried
Brains are not quite sealed
Brains are scrambled
Brat
Breakdown (e.g., mental, nervous)
Brokenhearted
Broken spirited
Bubbles in the think tank
Buffoon
Bug
Bugged out
Buggy
Bughouse
Bugs
Bulimia
Bulimorexia
Burn out a bearing
Burnout

Bust down
Butterflies (e.g., have butterflies in
   one's stomach)

C

Cabin fever
Cacesthesia
Cacodemonia (a mania that causes a
   person to believe himself pos-
   sessed and controlled by an evil
   spirit)
Cacoethes
Candidate for Bedlam
Cannabism
Ca-razy
Cardiac neurosis
Carnalism
Carpet biter
Case (e.g., a difficult case; a mental
   case)
Castles in Spain
Catalepsy
Catatonia
Catatonic
Cave in
Cement nut
Certified
Chapped nerves
Character neurosis
Checked his brains at the door
Chemical dependency
Chemical person
Chemophobia
Child abuse
Chloralism
Chloroformism
Choromania
Chronic
Chronic factitious illness
Clod-pated
Clouded mind

Clouded perception
Cocainism
Cockamamie
Cockeyed
Coco
Coconuts
Codependent
Come unhinged
Coming apart at the seams
Compulsion neurosis
Confused
Conk out
Conked
Conky
Conniption fit
Convulsed
Coocoo
Coop-happy
Coot
Corned
Crack
Crack-brained
Crack the brain
Cracked
Cracked egg
Cracked nut
Cracked up
Cracked wit
Crackers
Crackpot
Crackpotty
Crap out
Crazed
Crazier than a bedbug
Crazier than a quilt
Crazier than a shithouse rat
Crazified
Crazy (e.g., crazy as a coot; as a fox;
   as a bedbug; as a latrine rat; as a
   loon; as hell; as the devil)
Crazy boob
Crazy cat

Crazy-nuts
Creep
Crestfallen
Cretin
Cretinism
Crock
Cross as two sticks
Cuckoo
Cycling (e.g., rapid cycling—refer-
    ring to alternating elation and de-
    pression)
Cyclothymia (a temperament charac-
    terized by cyclic alterations of
    mood between elation and depres-
    sion)

D

Dada
Daffy
Daffy dame
Daffy daughter (or darter)
Daffy in the second story
Daffydil
Daft
Damaged
Deceived
Deinstitutionalized (e.g., mental pa-
    tient)
Delirium
Delusion (of being dead; of being ill
    [hypochondriasis]; of grandeur
    [megalomania]; of having cancer;
    of persecution [paranoia]). Cf. Pho-
    bias
Delusional
Dementia
Dementia praecox
Demonianism
Demonism
Demonolatry
Dense

Dependency
Dependent personality
Depression
Derailed
Derangement
Dereism (a mode of thinking directed
    away from reality and toward fan-
    tasy without cognizance of ordi-
    nary rules of logic)
Despairing
Despirited
Deterioration
Deviance
Devoid of reason
Diabolepsy (a state in which a person
    believes he is possessed by a devil
    or has been endowed with super-
    natural powers)
Diabolism (belief in or worship of
    the devil)
Dicked in the nob
Dim as a Toc H lamp
Ding
Ding-a-ling
Dingbats
Dingbatty
Dingdong daffy
Dingdongy
Dingy
Dip
Dippy
Dippy bat
Dippy batty
Dippy dame
Dippy in the dream box
Dip shit
Dipso
Dipstick
Disassociation neurosis
Disease
Disorder
Disorganized

Disorientation

Dispirited

Dissociative

Dissociative reaction

Dissolute

Distemptered

Distracted

Distraught

Disturbance

Disturbed

Dizzard

Dizzell

Dizzy

Do a brodie

Doctor Doddypoll

Does not have all his buttons

Does not have both feet on the ground

Does not have both oars in the water

Does not have enough sense to come
  in out of the rain

Does not have his ducks in a row

Does not have his head screwed on
  tight

Does not have his sail in the wind

Dolt

Doltish

Don Juan syndrome

Donkey

Donut-holes

Doodle

Doolally tap

Dope

Dope fiend

Dopey

Dork

Dotard

Dotage

Dotty

Dotty in the crumpet

Down (e.g., he feels down)

Down-and-out

Down in the dumps

Down in the mouth

Drapetomania (mental disease of
  black slaves in the South, making
  them run away to freedom in the
  North)

Drive up the wall

Drivelling (e.g., drivelling fool)

Drug abuse
  addiction
  delirium
  dependence
  dysfunctional use
  harmful use
  hazardous use
  intoxication
  misuse
  psychoactive drug abuse
  substance abuse
  unsanctioned drug use

Drug freak

Druggie

Drunk (see also separate list, beginning on page 81)

Duck-fit

Dull

Dullard

Dull understanding

Dull-witted

Dumb as a beetle

Dumdum

Dumb-nutty

Dummy

Dunce

Dunder-head

Dunder-pate

Dweeb

Dying duck in a thunderstorm

Dysaesthesia Aethiopis (mental disease of black slaves manifested
  their lassitude, reluctance to work,
  and breaking the master's valuable possessions)

Dyscontrol
Dysfunction
Dysfunctional family
Dysphoria
Dysthymia (extreme anxiety and de-
    pression accompanied by obsession)
Dysthymic

E

Eat [one's] heart out
Eating disorder (anorexia, bulemia,
    bulimia)
Eccentric
Effort syndrome
Egregious
Elation
Electra complex
Elevator doesn't go all the way to the
    top
Elevator doesn't stop on the top floor
Emotional (e.g., disorder; fatigue; ill-
    ness; upset)
Empty plate
Emptyheaded
Endogenous depression
Enthusiasm (e.g., he is a religious en-
    thusiast)
Eonism (the adoption, by a male, of
    feminine mannerisms, clothing,
    etc.)
Epicenism (the state or quality of
    combining characteristics of both
    sexes)
Erethism
Erotomania
Estranged
Euphoria
Excitement
Exhibitionism
Extravagant
Extroversion

F

Factitial illness
Factitious illness
Faker
Falling apart
Fanatic
Far gone
Far out
Far side
Farcical
Fathead
Fatuous
Feeble-mindedness
Feeblo
Feeling hopeless
Fetishism
A few bricks short of a full load
A few quarts low
Fiend
Fierce
Fifty cards in the deck
Fifty cents on the dollar
Fig newton
Finished (e.g., as in, He is finished)
Fit to be tied
Fits (e.g., has fits, fit for a madhouse,
    nuthouse, loony bin, etc.)
Fizz out
Flake
Flaky
Flathead
Flawed
Flighty
Flip one's lid
Flipped his lid
Flipped his wig
Flipped out
Flutter the dovecotes
Flying (e.g., he is flying)
Folly

Food addict (bulemic, bulimic, foodaholic)
Food for squirrels
Foofoo
Fool
Foolishness
Fool's paradise
Footy
Foxed
Fracture one's wig
Fracture one's toupee
Frantic
Frayed nerves
Freak out
Freaked out
Freaky
Frenzy (frenzied)
Fricked up
Frigidity
Frivolity
Fruit
Fruitcake (e.g., also, as in, nuttier than a fruitcake)
Fruitloops
Fruity
Fucked up (all fucked up; his/her mind is fucked up)
Fugue
Fugue state
Full of beans
Full of hops
Full of it
Full of nuts
Full of nuts as a fruitcake
Full of nuts as a peach-orchard boar
Full of nuts as a peanut bar
Full of shit
Funny
Funny-farm (e.g., fugitive from a funny-farm)
Funny farmer
Furor (furious)

Fury (excitement, mania)
Fussy as a hen with one chick
Fuzzy (e.g., fuzzy-headed)

G

Gabby
Ga-ga
Garret unfurnished
Gears are stripped
Geed up
Geeks
Geezed up
Georgia cracker
Get out of commission
Get out of gear
Get out of kelter (kilter)
Get out of whack
Get the wind up
Get up on the wrong side of the bed
Get wrong numbers
Get wrong orders from headquarters
Giddy
Giddybrain
Giggyhead
Giddypate
Gloomy Gus
Go ape
Go ausgespielt
Go balmy
Go bananas
Go batty
Go blooey
Go bung
Go flooey
Go haywire
Go into mental bankruptcy
Go off; Go off one's base
Go off one's bean
Go off one's chump
Go off one's head
Go off one's nut

Go off one's onion
Go off one's rocker
Go off the deep end
Go off the hooks
Go off the rail
Go off the track
Go off the trolley
Go on the blink
Go on the fritz
Go on the kibosh
Go on the rocks
Go pffft (or phut)
Go round the bend
Go to Battersea, to be cut for the simples
Go to pieces
Go to pot
Go to seed
Go wacky
Going to Springfield
Gomer (get out of my emergency room)
Gone
Gone ape
Gone astray
Gone bye-bye
Gone fishing
Gone haywire
Gone pffft (or phut)
Gone to pot
Goof
Goofball
Goofified
Goof-nuts
Goof-off
Goofy
Gooks
Goonybird
Goose
Got a lot on his mind
Got wrong orders from headquarters
Got too much on his mind

Got problems
Grandiosity (megalomania)
Guest in the attic
Guilt-Ridden

H

Habit (short for drug habit, or "he has a habit")
Haggard
Half-baked
Half-there
Half-witted
Hallucination
Hallucinosis
Hapless
Harum-scarum
Has a button missing
Has a hole in one's wig
Has a leak in the think tank
Has a problem
Has a vacant attic
Has a vacant belfry
Has a vacant garret
Has a vacant loft
Has a vacant top (or upper) story
Has no sense of proportion
Has rooms to rent
Has space to rent
Have a crack-up
Have a miss in one's motor
Have a moonflaw in the brain
Have a noise under one's hood
Have a screw loose
Have a slate loose
Have a smash-up
Have a tile loose
Have a worm in [one's] tongue
Have bats in [one's] belfry
Have kittens
Have one's attic unfurnished
Have sticky valves

Have windmills in [one's] head
Haywire
Head in the clouds
Head of wax
Head up his ass
Hebephrenia
Hebetude (the state, condition, or
    quality of being dull, enervated,
    or lethargic)
Heeby-jeebies
Heeled over
Herded one band of sheep too many
High (e.g., high as a kite)
High-strung
Hipped
Hippophile (a lover of horses)
Histriconism
Histrionicism
Hoboism
Hocky puck
Hoddy-doddy
Hole in the head (e.g., has a hole in
    his head)
Homeless (e.g., mental patient)
Homeless mentally ill
Homoeroticism
Honk out
Hooked
Hooliganism
Hopeless
Horrors (e.g., as in, He has the hor-
    rors)
Hospital addiction
Hospital hoboes
Hospital vagrants
Hospitalism
Humming bird
Hyped-up
Hyper
Hyperactive
Hyperactive child (Attention deficit
    disorder)

Hypersexuality
Hypochondriacism
Hypochondriasis
Hysteria
Hysterical
Hysteroepilepsy
Hysteropathy

I

Iatrogenic illness
Iatrogenic neurosis
Iconolatry (the worship or adoration
    of images)
Idiocy
Idiot
Idiotism
Ignoramus
Ill humored
Illness
Illogical
Illusive
Imaginary illness
Imbecility
Immaturity
Impossible
Impotence
Impulsive personality
Impulsivity
In a flap
In a lather
In a stew
In bad humor
In cuckoo-land
In low spirits
In never-never land
In the doldrums
In the dumps
In the ozone
Incapacity
Incompetence
Inebriated

Infantilism
Inferiority
Inferiority complex
Insanity
  Acute, confusional i.
  Adolescent i.
  Alcoholic i.
  Alternating i.
  Amenorrhoeal i.
  Apathic i.
  Atheromatous i.
  Certifiable i.
  Circular i.
  Climacteric i.
  Communicated i.
  Cyanotic i.
  Cyclic i.
  Delusional i.
  Deuteropathic i.
  Dissolute i.
  Dodge i.
  Homicidal i.
  Hysterical i.
  Ideal i.
  Idiopathic i.
  Impulsive i.
  Incurable i.
  Induced i.
  Insanity of childhood i.
  Insanity of negation i.
  Insanity of pregnancy i.
  Intellectual i.
  Intelligential i.
  Involute i.
  Legal i.
  Masturbational i.
  Masturbatory i.
  Melancholic i.
  Moral i.
  Notional i.
  Old maid's i.
  Ovarian i.

  Periodic i.
  Permanent i.
  Presenile i.
  Progressive systematized i.
  Protopathic i.
  Psychic i.
  Psychocerebral i.
  Pubescent i.
  Puerperal i.
  Reasoning i.
  Saturnine i.
  Secondary i.
  Sequelar i.
  Stuporous i.
  Symptomatic i.
  Syphilitic i.
  Temporary i.
  Toxic i.
  Uterine i.
  Volitional i.
Insensate
Insulse
Intoxicated
Introversion
Invalidism
Inversion
Irrationality
Irresponsibility (e.g., he is not respon-
  sible (by reason of insanity)
Itarogenic neurosis
Ithyphallicism (the worship of an
  erect phallus or the use of a repre-
  sentation of one in ritual)

J

Jambled
Jammed
Jeepy
Jesus freak
Jiggered up
Jimjams

Jimmed up
Jinglebrains
Just plain nuts

K

Kaput
Keyed up Kink in the conk
Klepto
Kleptomania
Knock for a loop
Kook
Kooky

L

Lacks
Lacks all sense of proportion
Lacks good judgment
Lacks good sense
Lamebrain
Larrikinism (the state of being noisy,
    rowdy, or disorderly)
Leak in the think tank
Lemon flake
Lesbianism
Lexical-syntactic disorder
Light's on but nobody's home
Like a bear with a sore head
Like a cat in a strange garret
Like a cat on a hot tin roof
Like a chicken with its head cut off
Listless
Litigious (e.g., paranoid)
Litigiousness
A little off plumb
A little slow
A little touched
Loco
Locoed
Looby
Loon

Loony (e.g., loony bird)
Loony-tick
Loony-tunes
Loopy
Loose in the bean
Loose in the hilts
Loose in the nut
Loose in the upper story
Loose nut
Loose-nutty
Loose on the top
Loose screw
Lose one's bearings
Lose one's head
Lose one's marbles
Lose one's taffy
Lost
Lost all sense of proportion
Lost his faculties
Lost his head
Lost his marbles
Lost his mind
Low (e.g., feeling low)
Low pilot light
Low self esteem
Lunacy
Lunatic
Lunatic fringe
Luny
Lycanthropy

M

Mad (e.g., a mad dog; mad as a hat-
    ter; as a baited bull; as a buck; as
    a cut snake; as a hatter; as hops;
    as a maggot; as a March hare; as
    May butter; as a meat-axe; as
    mud; as a tup; as a weaver; as a
    wet hen)
Mad-brained
Madcap

Mad dog
Mad Greek
Mad haddock
Mad hatter
Mad Tom (also Tom of Bedlam, in
    the seventeenth century a rogue
    who feigned madness)
Madman
Madness
Maenadism (behavior characteristic
    of a maenad or bacchante; raging
    or wild behavior in a woman)
Malady
Maladjustment
Malignant narcissism
Malingering (to feign insanity)[11]
    Crown a Napoleon
    Do a Brody
    Play the squirrel
    Put on a circus
    Put on the balmy stick
    Throw an ingbing
    Throw a wingding
    Turn a cartwheel
    Work one's ticket
Mania(s) (an infatuation with, abnor-
    mal love of, obsession with, or
    passion for . . .; e.g., kleptomania,
    etc.)

Manias

List 1[12]

acromania (violent mania; incurable
    insanity)
agoramania (m. for open spaces)
agyiomania (m. for streets)
ailuromania (l. of cats)
alcoholomania (l. of alcohol)
amaxomania (m. for being in vehicles)
amenomania (m. for pleasing delu-
    sions)

Americamania (i. with America and
    things American)
andromania (i. with men; cf. nympho-
    mania)
aphrodisiomania (m. for sexual plea-
    sure)
apimania (l. of bees)
automania (l. of solitude)
autophonomania (i. with suicide)
ballistomania (i. with bullets)
bibliomania (l. of books)
cheromania (l. of gaiety)
Chinamania (i. with China and things
    Chinese)
chionomania (m. for snow)
choreomania (m. for dancing)
chrematomania (m. for money)
clinomania (m. for bed rest)
coporolalomania (m. for foul speech)
cremnomania (i. with cliffs)
cresomania (m. for great wealth)
cynomania (l. of dogs)
Dantomania (m. for Dante and his
    works)
demomania (ochlomania)
demonomania (a monomania in
    which a person believes he is pos-
    sessed of devils; also called
    demonopathy)
doramania (m. for fur)
drapetomania (m. for running away)
dromomania (m. for travel)
ecdemiomania (m. for wandering)
edeomania (o. with genitals)
egomania (egotism)
empleomania (o. with public employ-
    ment)
enomania (m. for wine; also called
    oinomania)
entheomania (m. for religion)
entomomania (l. of insects)
eremiomania (m. for stillness)

ergasiomania (m. for activity)

ergomania (m. for work; also called workaholic)

eroticomania (o. with erotica)

erotographomania (o. with erotic literature)

erotomania (preoccupation with sexual desire, often for a celebrity or other relative stranger)

erythromania (m. for blushing)

etheromania (m. for ether)

florimania (m. for plants and flowers)

Francomania (o. with France and things French)

gamomania (m. characterized by strange and extravagant proposals of marriage; excessive longing for the married state)

gephyromania (m. for crossing bridges)

Germanomania (o. with Germany and things German; also called Teutonomania)

graphomania (o. with writing)

Grecomania (o. with Ancient Greece and Greeks)

hymnomania (m. for nakedness)

gynecomania (o. with sexual desire for women)

hamartomania (o. with sin)

hedonomania (m. for pleasure)

heliomania (l. of the sun)

hieromania (m. for priests)

hippomania (m. for horses)

hodomania (l. of travel)

homicidomania (m. for murder)

hydrodipsomania (l. of drinking water)

hydromania (l. of water)

hylomania (m. for wood)

hypermania (an acute mania)

hypnomania (m. for sleep)

hypomania (mild mania; submania)

hysteromania (nymphomania)

ichthyomania (l. of fish)

iconomania (m. for icons)

idolomania (m. for idols)

Italomania (o. with Italy and things Italian)

kainomania (m. for novelty)

Kathisomania (m. for sitting)

kinesomania (m. for movement)

lalomania (l. of speech or talking)

lethomania (m. for narcotics)

logomania (m. for words or talking; also called logorrhea)

lycomania (lycanthropy, insanity characterized by the person believing he is a wolf)

lypemania (tendency toward deep malancholy)

macromania (m. for becoming larger)

mania (manic-depressive psychosis; bipolar disorder; any excessive excitement or activity)

megalomania (grandiosity; conceit)

mentulomania (o. with the penis)

mesmeromania (o. with hypnosis)

micromania (m. for becoming smaller)

monomania (1. insanity confined to delusions confined to one idea or subject; excessive interest in or enthusiasm for a single thing or idea; obsession)

morphiomania (addiction to morphine)

musicomania (m. for music)

musomania (l. of mice)

mythomania (l. of myths)

narcomania (addiction to drugs, especially narcotics)

necromania (o. with death or the dead; cf. thanatomania)

noctimania (l. of the night)

nosomania (o. with imagined disease)

nostomania (homesickness; nostalgia)

nudomania (m. for nudity)

nymphomania (m. for frequent, continued sexual intercourse by a woman; also called oestromania; cf. satyromania)

ochlomania (m. for crowds; also called demomania)

oestromania (nymphomania)

oikomania (m. for one's home, for staying at home)

oinomania (m. for wine; also called enomania)

oligomania (m. confined to several subjects; cf. monomania)

oniomania (m. for buying articles of all kinds)

ophidiomania (l. of reptiles)

opiomania (addiction to opium)

opsomania (m. for special kinds of food; cf. phagomania, sitomania)

orchidomania (o. with testicles)

ornithomania (l. of birds)

paramania (l. of complaining)

parousiamania (o. with the second coming of Christ)

pathomania (moral insanity)

phagomania (m. for food and eating; cf. opsomania, sitomania)

phaneromania (m. for picking at growths)

pharmacomania (m. for drugs or medicines)

philopatridomania (homesickness)

phonomania (l. of noise)

photomania (l. of light)

phronemomnia (m. for thinking)

phthisiomania (o. with tuberculosis)

politicomania (m. for politics)

poriomania (ambulatory automatism; [unconscious] tendency to walk away from home)

pornographomania (m. for pornography)

potomania (l. of alcohol; alcoholism; delirium tremens; also called tromomania)

Russomania (o. with Russia and things Russian)

satyromania (m. for frequent, continued sexual intercourse in a man; cf. nymphomania)

scribomania (m. for writing)

sideromania (o. with railroad travel)

sitomania (o. with food; cf. phagomania, opsomania; bulemia)

sophomania (conviction of one's own wisdom)

squandermania (m. for spending money)

submania (mild mania; hypomania)

symmetromania (m. for symmetry)

Teutonomania (Germanomania)

thalassomania (l. of the sea)

thanatomania (o. with death; cf. necromania)

theatromania (m. for the theater)

timbromania (m. for postage stamps)

tomomania (o. with surgery)

trichomania (o. with hair)

trichorrhexomania (m. for pinching off one's hair)

tristimania (melancholia; depression)

tromomania (delirium tremens; also called potomania)

Turkomania (o. with Turkey and things Turkish)

typomania (o. with the expectation of publication)

uteromania (nymphomania)

xenomania (m. for foreigners)

zoomania (l. of animals)

List 2

mania, absorbed (manic stupor)

acute

akinetic (motionless)

ambitious

a potu (alcoholic)

Bell's (acute)

brooding

Caesar (megalomania)

chattering

chronic

chronic intellectual

collecting

concionabunda (m. for addressing the public)

dancing

doubting mania (morbid scrupulosity in regard to minutiae)

ephemeral

errabunda (m. for impulsive wandering)

grumbling

homicidal

incendiary (pyromania)

inhibited

metaphysical (insanity of doubt)

mitis (hypomania)

phantastica infantilis (confabulation in children)

peracute mania (acute maniacal excitement)

puerperal mania (puerperal psychosis; postpartum psychosis; acute mental disorder in women after childbirth)

reactive

religious

senilis

sine delirio (without delirium)

stuporous

transitoria

wandering

Maniac

Maniaphobia (fear of insanity)

Manic

Manipulative

March to the beat of a different drummer

Masturbation (onanism, self-abuse)

Masturbatory insanity

Masturbatory orgasmic inadequacy

Mattoid

Mean as hungry Tyson (Australian phrase)

Meet [one's] Waterloo

Megalomania (delusion of grandeur, grandiosity)

Melancholia

Melancholian

Melancholy

Mental(e.g., case; disorder; disease; illness; sickness, wreck)

Mental aberration

Mental agitation

Mental alienation

Mental anorexia

Mental auto-infection

Mental disease

Mental disorder

Mental illness

Mental vacation

Mentally bankrupt

Mentally deranged

Mentally finished

Mentally kaput

Mentally ruined

Mentally unsound

Mentally wrecked

Merycism (a condition in which food is chewed, . . . swallowed, and then returned to the mouth and chewed again)

Meshuga

Messed-Up

Midsummer madness

Milky in the filbert

Mind is spent (e.g., shot, gone, blown)

Mindless
Minus some buttons
Misguided
Misled
Misocainea (an abnormal dislike for new ideas)
Miss Nancy
Miss one's buttons
Miss one's marbles
Miss something upstairs
Miss the boat
Mixed pathology
Mixed personality disorder
Mixed up
Mokus (crazy thinking even when sober; used by alcoholics)
Monoideism (the focusing of the attention on a single thing, especially as a result of hypnosis)
Monomania
Mood disorder
Moody
Moonrakers
Moon-struck
Moron
Moronic
Moronism
Morosity
Morphinism
Muddled
Muddle-headed
Multiple (short for multiple personality)
Multiple personality
Munchausen syndrome
Mushroom eater
Mutt
Muttonhead

N

Narcissism
Narcolepsy

Narcoleptic
Narcosynthesis
Narcoticism
Necrosadism
Needs a checkup from the neck up
Needs a rest
Needs help
Needs his head examined
Nerts
Nertsy
Nertz
Nertzy
Nerves
Nervous (e.g., breakdown; disease; he's got a bad case of nerves)
Nervous exhaustion
Neurasthenia
Neurocirculatory asthenia
Neuropsychiatric (e.g., case, disability)
Neurosis
Neurosism
Neurosismus
Neurosyphilis
Neurotic antithesis
    anxiety
    depression
    dissociation
    personality
Neuroticism
Nicotine dependence
Nicotinism
Nincompoop
Ninny
Nitwit
Nizy
No beans in the pod
No brains (e.g., he has no brains)
No joy in Mudville
No kernels in the nut
No milk in the coconut
No one at home

No seeds in the pod
No seeds in the pumpkin
Nobody at home
Nobody home in the upper story
Non compos
Non compos mentis
Noncomformist
Noodle
Noodlehead
Not all there
Not bright
Not cooking on all burners
Not functioning in all circuits
Not have all [one's] buttons
Not in possession of all his faculties
Not playing with a full deck
Not quite right
Not right
Not running on all cylinders
Not to know if [one] is afoot or on
    horseback
Not to know if [one] is coming or
    going
Not to know which end is up
Not together
Not too swift
Not well put together
Not wrapped tight
Numskull
Nut
Nuts
Nuts and bolts
Nutsy
Nutty (e.g., also, as in, nuttier than a
    fruitcake)
Nutty as a chinkapin
Nutty as a fruitcake
Nutty as a peanut bar
Nutwit
Nutwitted
Nutzo
Nympho

Nympholepsy (an ecstatic variety of
    demonic possession believed by
    the ancients to be inspired by
    nymphs)
Nymphomania

O

Oaf
Odd
Oddball
Onanism
Obsessional neurosis
Obtuse
Odd
Oddball
Oedipus complex
Off
Off at the nail
Off his rocker
Off his trolley
Off in the upper story
Off one's base
Off one's bean
Off one's box
Off one's chump
Off one's head
Off one's kerbase
Off one's nut
Off one's onion
Off one's rails
Off one's rocker
Off one's track
Off one's trolley
Off the beam
Off the bean
Off the deep end (e.g., gone off the
    deep end)
Off the hinges
Off the map
Off the nut
Off the wall

Offbeat

-oholic (abnormally interested in, addicted to-)
   alcoholic
   bookaholic
   chocaholic
   foodaholic (bulemic)
   lovaholic
   musicaholic
   sexaholic
   workaholic

On his top

On the blink

On the fritz

On the kibosh

On the rack

On the rocks

Onanism (masturbation, self-abuse)

Onchyphagia (nailbiting)

One brick short of a full load

Opiophagism

Opiophobia

Opiumism

Organia

Organic mental illness

Organic psychosis

Organic-toxic psychosis

Orgasmic inadequacy

Ork-orks

Out in left field

Out in left field and everyone else is
   playing football

Out in space

Out in the rain too long

Out in the sun too long

Out of commish

Out of commission

Out of control

Out of countenance

Out of funds

Out of gear

Out of his gourd

Out of his head

Out of his mind

Out of his nut

Out of his onion

Out of his tree

Out of his wits

Out-of-it

Out of key

Out of kilter (kelter)

Out of order

Out of sorts

Out of touch

Out of town

Out of whack

Out to lunch

Overwrought

Owl

P

Palooka

Panic disorder

Paralogia

Paralyzed

Paramnesia (a distortion of memory
   in which fact and fantasy are confused)

Paranoia

Paranoid

Paranoidism

Passive-aggressive

Patchy

Pathological (e.g., gambling, mourn-
   ing)

Pathomimia

Pea-brain

A peg too low

Pension neurosis

Peregrinating patients

Perversion

Peter Pan Syndrome

Phantasmagored

Pharmacothymia (drug addiction)

Philauty (self love; an excessive regard for oneself)

Philia(s) (abnormal love of, or passion for, an idea, thing or person; often accompanied by a desire to collect the object)

aileurophilia, ailurophilia (l. of cats)

algophilia (l. of pain)

Anglophile (l. of England and things English)

audiophile (l. of high-fidelity sound equipment and recordings on tape or disks)

audiophilia (the condition of an audiophile; the state of one who listens to high-fidelity equipment solely for the quality of reproduction)

autophilia (self-love; narcissism)

bibliophilia (l. of books)

carcinophilia (affinity of certain chemical agents for cancerous tissue)

cinephilia (l. of moviegoing)

claustrophilia (l. of closed spaces, of being indoors)

coprophilia (l. of obscenity; an abnormal interest in feces, especially as a source of sexual excitement; the use of obscene or scatological language fors sexual gratification)

demophilia (l. of crowds)

discophily, diskophily (l. of studying and collecting phonograph records; also called phonophily)

Francophilia (l. of France and things French)

galeophilia (aileurophilia)

Germanophilia (l. of Germany and things German)

Gerontophilia (sexual attraction to the elderly)

gramophilia (l. of phonograph records)

hydrophily (an affinity for water, a property of certain materials)

iconophiliia (l. of pictures, prints, engravings, lithographs)

laparotomaphilia (l. of abdominal surgery)

musicophilia (l. of music)

mysophilia (l. of filth)

mythophilia (l. of myths)

necrophilia (necrophily, necrophilism; erotic attraction to corpses)

nemophilia (l. of forests and woods)

nosophilia (l. of being ill; malingering; also called pathophilia)

nyctophilia (l. of the night, in preference to the day)

paraphilia (perversion; engaging in abnormal sexual activities)

pathophilia (nosophilia)

pharmacophilia (pharmacothymia; drug addiction)

phonophilia (discophilia)

pyrophilia (l. of fire)

Russophilia (l. of Russia and things Russian)

scopophilia (passive scopophilia: sexual pleasure from viewing nude bodies, sexual acts, or erotic photographs; active scopophilia: sexual excitement or pleasure from being seen nude; exhibitionism)

Slavophiliia (l. of Slavs and things Slavic)

taphophilia (l. of funerals, graves, and cemeteries)

toxophilia (l. of archery)

traumatophilia (l. of injuries, wounds)

zoophilia (l. of animals; desire for sexual activity with animals; zoophilism, zoophily)

Phobia(s) (excessive aversion to, or
   abnormal, excessive, or morbid
   fear of...)

Phobias

List 1[14]

acarophobia (f. of skin infestation by
   mites or ticks)
acerophobia (f. of sourness)
achluophobia (scotophobia)
acidophobia (inability to accommo-
   date to acid soils, as certain plants)
acousticophobia (f. of noise)
acrophobia (f. of heights; also called
   altophobia, batophobia, hypsophobia)
aelurophobia (ailurophobia)
aerophobia (f. of drafts; cf. ancraophobia, anemophobia)
agoraphobia (f. of being in crowded,
   public places, like markets; cf.
   demophobia)
agyrophobia (f. of crossing streets;
   also dromophobia)
aichmophobia, aichurophobia (f. of
   pointed objects)
AIDS phobia
ailurophobia, aelurophobia, elurophobia (f. of cats; also called gatophobia, felinophobia)
akoustikophobia (f. of sound)
albuminurophobia (f. of albumin in
   one's urine as a sign of kidney disease)
algophobia (f. of pain; cf. odynophobia)
altophobia, acrophobia (f. of heights)
amathophobia (f. of dust)
amaxophobia (f. of being or riding in
   vehicles)
ancraophobia (f. of wind; cf. aerophobia, anemophobia)

androphobia (1. f. of men; 2. hatred
   of males; cf. gynephobia)
anemophobia (f. of drafts or winds;
   cf. aerophobia, ancraophobia)
anginophobia (f. of quinsy or other
   forms of sore throat)
Anglophobia (a hatred or f. of England and things English)
anthophobia (f. of flowers)
anthropophobia (f. of people, especially in groups)
antlophobia (f. of floods)
apeirophobia (f. of infinity)
aphephobia (f. of touching or being
   touched; also called haphephobia,
   haptephobia, thixophobia)
apiphobia, apiophobia (f. of bees;
   also called melissophobia)
arachnephobia (f. of spiders)
asthenophobia (f. of weakness)
astraphobia, astrapophobia (f. of
   lightning; cf. brontophobia,
   keraunophobia)
astrophobia (siderophobia)
ataxiophobia, ataxophobia (f. of disorder, of falling)
atelophobia (f. of imperfection)
atephobia (f. of ruin)
aulophobia (f. of flutes)
aurophobia (a. to gold)
automysophobia (f. being dirty; cf.
   misophobia)
autophobia, autophoby (f. of being
   by oneself, of solitude; also called
   eremiophobia, eremophobia,
   monophobia)
bacillophobia (f. of germs; also
   called bacteriophobia)
ballistophobia (f. of missiles)
barophobia (f. of gravity)
basiphobia (f. of walking; also called
   bathmophobia)

bathophobia (f. of depth; a. to bathing)

batophobia (f. of passing high buildings; acrophobia)

batrachophobia (f. of frogs and toads)

belonephobia (f. of pins and needles)

bibliophobia (a. to books)

blennophobia (f. of slime; also called myxophobia)

bogyphobia (f. of demons and goblins)

bromidrosiphobia (f. of having a bad body odor)

brontophobia (f. of thunder and thunderstorms; also called tonitrophobia; cf. astraphobia, keraunophobia)

cainophobia (f. of novelty; also called cainotophobia, neophobia)

carcinomophobia, carcinomatophobia, carcinophobia (f. of cancer; also called cancerophobia)

cardiophobia (f. of heart disease)

cathisophobia (f. of sitting down)

catoptrophobia (f. of mirrors)

Celtophobia (a. to Celts)

cenophobia, kenophobia (f. of a void or of open spaces)

ceraunophobia (keraunophobia)

chaetophobia (f. of hair)

cheimaphobia, cheimatophobia (f. of cold; cf. cryophobia, psychrophobia)

chemophobia (f. of chemical contamination of the environment)

cherophobia (f. of gaiety)

chinophobia (f.of, a. to, snow)

cholerophobia (f. of cholera)

chrematophobia (f. of wealth)

chromatophobia (f. of colors)

chrometophobia (f. of money)

chromophobia (f. of colors)

chronophobia (f. of time, of having to be on time)

cibophobia (f. of food; also called sitophobia, sitiophobia; cf. phagophobia)

claustrophobia (f, of enclosed spaces; also called cleistophobia)

cleptophobia (kleptophobia)

clinophobia (f. of going to bed)

clithrophobia (an abnormal fear of enclosed spaces)

coitophobia (f. of coitus; also called genophobia; cf. erotophobia)

cometophobia (f. of comets)

computerphobia (f. of computers)

coprophobia (f. of excrement)

cremnophobia (f. of precipices)

cryophobia (f. of ice or frost; cf. cheimaphobia)

crystallophobia (f. of glass; also called hyalophobia)

cymophobia (f. of waves)

cynophobia (f. of dogs; cf. kynophobia)

cypridophobia (f. of venereal disease; also called venereophobia)

deipnophobia (f. of dining and dinner conversation)

demonophobia (f. of demons)

demophobia (f. of crowds)

dermatophobia (f. of skin disease; also called dermatosiophobia, dermatopathophobia)

dextrophobia (f. of objects on the right side of the body; cf. levophobia)

diabetophobia (f. of diabetes)

dikephobia (f. of justice)

dinophobia (f. of whirlpools)

diplopiaphobia (f. of double vision)

dipsophobia (f. of drinking, esp. alcohol)

domatophobia (f. of being in a house)

doraphobia (f. of fur)

dromophobia (agoraphobia; kinetophobia)

dysmorphophobia (f. of deformity, usually in others; also called dysmorphobia, dysmorphomania)

ecclesiophobia (f. of the church)

ecophobia, oecophobia, oikophobia (a. to home surroundings)

eisoptrophobia (f. of mirrors)

electrophobia (f. of electricity)

eleutherophobia (f. of freedom)

elurophobia (ailurophobia)

emetophobia (f. of vomiting)

enetophobia (f. of needles)

entomophobia (f. of insects)

eosophobia (f. of the dawn)

eremiophobia, eremophobia (autophobia)

ereuthophobia (f. of blushing)

ergasiophobia (a. to work; also called ergophobia)

erotophobia (f. of sexual arousal and feelings and their physical expression; also called miserotica; cf. coitophobia)

erythrophobia (f. of the color red; f. of blushing)

eurotophobia (f. of female genitals)

febriphobia (f. of fever)

felinophobia (ailurophobia)

Francophobia, Gallophobia (a. to France or things French)

galeophobia (f. of sharks)

Gallophobia (Francophobia)

gametophobia, gamophobia (f. of, marriage)

gatophobia (ailurophobia)

genophobia (coitophobia)

gephyrophobia (f. of crossing a bridge)

gerascophobia (f. of growing old)

Germanophobia (a. to Germany, or things German; also called Teutophobia, Teutonophobia)

geumatophobia, geumophobia (f. of tastes or flavors; cf. olfactophobia)

glossophobia (f. of speaking in public or of trying to speak)

graphophobia (a. to writing)

gringophobia (in Spain or Latin America, a. to white strangers, especialy to people from the United States)

gymophobia (f. of nudity; also called nudophobia)

gynephobia, gynophobia (f.of women; cf. androphobia, parthenophobia)

hadephobia (f. of hell; also called stygiophobia)

haemaphobia (hemophobia)

hagiophobia (a. to saints and the holy)

hamartophobia (f. of error or sin)

haphephobia, haphophobia, haptephobia, haptophobia (aphephobia; also called thixophobia)

harpaxophobia (f. of robbers; cf. kleptophobia)

hedonophobia (f. of pleasure; also called anhedonia)

heliophobia (a. to, or f. of, sunlight)

helminthophobia (f. of being infested with worms; cf. scoleciphobia)

hemaphobia, haemaphobia, hemophibia (f. of the sight of blood; also called hematophobia)

herpetophobia (f. of reptiles; cf. ophidiophobia)

hierophobia (f. of sacred objects)

hippophobia (f. of horses)

hodophobia (fear of travel)

homichlophobia (f. of fog)

homilophobia (a. to sermons)

homophobia (a. to or f. of homosexuality; cf. uranophobia)

hyalophobia (crystallophobia)

hydrophobia (f. of water; also a symptom of, and name for, rabies)

hydrophobophobia (f. of rabies; also called lyssophobia; cf. kynophobia)

hygrophobia (f. of liquids in any form, especially wine and water)

hylephobia (a. to wood or woods)

hypegiaphobia, hypengyophobia (f. of responsibility; cf. paraliopophobia)

hypnophobia (f. of sleep)

hypsophobia, hypsiphobia (acrophobia)

iatrophobia (f. of doctors, of going to the doctor)

ichthyophobia (f.of fish)

iconophobia (f. of icons)

ideophobia (f. of ideas)

iophobia (f. of poisons; cf. toxiphobia)

isopterophobia (f. of termites)

Judophobia (a. to Jews and of Jewish culture; also called Judosphobism, Judaeophobia, anti-Semitism)

kakorrhaphiophobia (f. of failure or defeat)

katagelophobia (f. of ridicule)

kenophobia (f. open spaces)

keraunophobia, ceraunophobia (f. of thunder and lightning; cf. astraphobia, brontophobia)

kinetophobia (f. of motion; also called dromophobia)

kleptophobia, cleptophobia (f. of thieves or of the loss through thievery; cf. harpaxophobia)

kopophobia (f. of mental or physical exhaustion)

kynophobia, cynophobia (f. of psuedorabies; cf. hydrophobophobia)

laliophobia, lalophobia (f. of talking)

lepraphobia (f. of leprosy)

levophobia (f. of objects on the left side of the body; cf. dextrophobia)

limnophobia (f. of lakes)

linonophobia (f. of string)

logophobia (f. of words)

lyssophobia (f. of becoming insane; cf. hydrophobophobia)

maieusiophobia (tocophobia)

maniaphobia (f. of madness)

mastigophobia (f. of being beaten)

mechanophobia (f. of machinery)

melissophobia (apiphobia)

meningitophobia (f. of miningitis)

merinthophobia (f. of being bound or restrained)

metallophobia (f. of metals)

meteorophobia (f. of meteors or meteorites)

microbiophobia (f. of bacteria or microbes)

misophobia, musophobia, mysophobia (f. of dirt, especially of being contaminated by dirt; cf. automysophobia, rhypophobia)

molysomophobia (f. of infection)

monopathophobia (f. of sickness in a crtain part of the body)

monophobia (autophobia)

motorphobia (f. of motor vehicles)

musicophobia (a. to music)

musophobia (f. of mice; cf. misophobia)

mysophobia (misophobia)

mythophobia (a. to myths; f. of making false statements)

myxophobia (blennophobia)

necrophobia (f. of death and of corpses; also called thanatophobia)

negrophobia (a. to Negroes)

neophobia (cainophobia)

nephophobia (f. of clouds)

noctiphobia (f. of the night; cf. nyctophobia)

nomatophobia (f. of names)

nosophobia (f. of contracting disease)

nudophobia, nudiphobia (gymnophobia)

nyctophobia (f. of darkness or night; cf. noctiphobia)

ochlophobia (f. of crowds)

ochophobia (f. of vehicles)

odontophobia (f. of teeth, especially those of animals)

odynophobia (f. of pain; cf. algophobia)

oenophobia, oinophobia (a. to wine)

oikophobia (f. of home surroundings)

olfactophobia (a. to smells; also called osmophobia, osphresiophobia; cf. geumophobia)

ombrophobia (f. of rain)

ommatophobia (f. of eyes)

onomatophobia (f. of a certain name)

ophidiophobia (f. of snakes; also called ophiophobia; cf. herpetophobia)

opiophobia (f. by physician of prescribing opium, opioid analgesics, or any controlled analgesic)

ornithophobia (f. of birds)

osmophobia (olfactophobia)

osphresiophobia (olfactophobia)

ouranophobia (uranophobia)

paedophobia (pedophobia)

panophobia (a state of general anxiety; f. of everything; also panphobia, pantaphobia, pantophobia)

papaphobia (a. to the pope or the papacy)

paralipophobia (f. of neglecting some duty; cf. hypengyophobia)

paraphobia (f. of sexual perversion)

parasitophobia (f. of parasites)

parthenophobia (a. to young girls; cf. gynephobia)

pathophobia (f. of disease)

peccatiphobia, peccatophobia (f. of sinning)

pediculophobia (f. of lice; also called phthiriophobia)

pediophobia (a. to children)

pedophobia, paedophobia (a. to dolls)

pellagraphobia (f. of pellagra)

peniaphobia (f. of poverty)

phagophobia (f. of eating; cf. anorexia)

pharmacophobia (f. of drugs)

phasmophobia (f. of ghosts; cf. pneumatophobia, spectrophobia)

phengophobia (f. of daylight)

philosophobia (a. to philosophy or philosophers)

phobophobia (f. of fear itself)

phonophobia (f. of noise or loud talking)

photalgiophobia (f. of photalgia, pain in the eyes caused by light)

photophobia (f. of light; painful sensitivity to light; also called photodysphoria; tendency to thrive in reduced light, as exhibited by certain plants)

phronemophobia (f. of thinking)

phthiriophobia (pediculophobia)

phthisiophobia (f. of tuberculosis; also called tuberculophobia)

pneumatophobia (f. of incorporeal beings, ghosts; cf. phasmophobia, spectrophobia)

pnigophobia (f. of choking)

pogonophobia (a. to beards)

poinephobia (f. of punishment)

politicophobia (a. to politicians)

polyphobia (f. of many things; cf. panophobia)

ponophobia (f. of fatigue, especially through overworking)

potamophobia (f. of rivers)

proctophobia (apprehension in patients with a rectal disease)

proteinphobia (a. to protein-containing foods)

psychophobia (f. of the mind)

psychrophobia (f. of the cold; cf. cheimaphobia)

pteronophobia (f. of feathers)

pyrexiophobia (f. of fever; cf. thermophobia)

pyrophobia (f. of fire)

rhabdophobia (f. of being beaten; f. of magic)

rhypophobia (f. of filth; cf. misophobia)

Russophobism, Russophobia (a. to Russians and things Russian)

Satanophobia (f. of Satan)

scabiophobia (f. of scabies)

scatophobia (f. of using obscene language; coprophobia)

sciophobia (f. of shadows)

scoleciphobia (f. of worms; also called vermiphobia; cf. helminthophobia)

scopophobia (f. of being looked at; also scoptophobia)

scotophobia (f. of the dark; also called achluophobia)

selaphobia (f. of flashes of light)

siderodromophobia (f. of railroads or of traveling on trains)

siderophobia (f. of the stars; also called astrophobia)

sitophobia, sitiophobia (cibophobia)

Slavophobia (a. to things Slavic, especially to their real or imagined political influence)

spectrophobia (f. of specters or phantoms; cf. phasmophobia, pneumatophobia)

stasibasiphobia (f. of not being able to stand or walk; f. of attempting to do either)

stasiphobia, stasophobia (f. of standing upright)

stygiophobia (hadephobia)

symmetrophobia (f. of symmetry)

syphiliphobia, syphilophobia (f. of having or becoming infected with syphilis; cf. cypridophobia)

tabophobia (f. of a wasting sickness)

tachophobia (f. fear of speed)

taphephobia, taphiphobia, taphophobia (f. of being buried alive)

tapinophobia (f. of small things)

taurophobia (f. of bulls)

teleophobia (a. to teleology)

telephononphobia (f. of using the telephone)

teratophobia (f. of monsters or of giving birth to a monster)

Teutophobia, Teutonophobia (Germanophobia)

thaasophobia (f. of being idle)

thalassophobia (f. of the sea)

thanatophobia (necrophobia)

theatrophobia (f. of theaters)

theophobia (f. of God)

thermophobia (f. of heat; cf. pyrexiophobia)

thixophobia (aphephobia)

tocophobia, tokophobia (f. of childbirth; also called maieusiophobia)

tomophobia (f. of surgical operations)

tonitrophobia, tonitruphobia (brontophobia)

topophobia (f. of certain places)

toxiphobia, toxicophobia (f. of being poisoned; cf. iophobia) traumatophobia (f. of war or physical injury)

tremophobia (f. of trembling)

trichinophobia (f. of trichinosis; also called trichophobia, trichopathophobia)

tridecaphobia (triskaidekaphobia)

triskaidekaphobia (f. of the number 13; also called tridecaphobia)

trypanophobia (vaccinophobia)

tuberculophobia (phthisiophobia)

tyrannophobia (f. of tyrants)

uranophobia (f. of homosexuals and homosexuality; homophobia; also fear of the heavens; ouranophobia)

urophobia (f. of passing urine)

accinophobia (f. of vaccines and vaccination; also called trypanophobia)

venereophobia (cypridophobia)

vermiphobia (scoleciphobia)

xenophobia (f. of foreigners and strange things)

zelophobia (f. of jealousy)

zoophobia (f. of animals)

List 2[15]

phobia,
    bathroom
    bug
    cancer
    death
    doorknob
    hypochondriacal
    impregnation
    infection
    insect
    landscape
    light-and-shadow
    live burial
    poisoning
    school
    social
    street
    toilet
    traumatic
    vehicle

Phonological-snytactic disorder

Pie in the sky

Piffed

Pifflicated

Pinhead

Pipe dream

Pixilated

Play goat

Play monkey

Play the fool

Played too long without a helmet

Playing with only half a deck

Playing with the squirrels

Plerophory

Plumb locoed

Poco loco

Polle syndrome

Polydemonism

Polysurgical addiction

Poor head

Poor stick

Popped his cork

Possessed

Possessed with the devil

Postpartum delirium

Postpartum psychosis

Post-traumatic (e.g., neurosis; stress disorder)

Potted

Potts (Italian)

Potty

Pretty fellow

Problem (e.g., has a problem)

Problem patients

Professional patients

Prune

Pseudomania

Psychalgia (mental or psychic pain)
Psychiatric (e.g., disease; disorder; disturbance)
Psycho
Psycho case
Psychoactive substance abuse
Psycholepsy
Psychopathology
Psychopathological
Psychopathy
Psychophobia
Psychosis
Psychosomatic
Puerile
Puerilism
Puerperal delirium
Puerperal psychosis
Pumpkin head
Putz
Pyromania

Q

Queer (e.g., applied especially to homosexuals)
Queer in the attic
Queer in the head
Queered
Quisby
Quixotism

R

Rabid
Rambling
Rash
Rats in the attic
Rats in the belfry
Rats in the garret
Rats in the upper story
Rattlebean

Rattlebrain
Rattlecap
Rattlehead
Rattlenut
Rattleskull
Ratty
Ratty as a jaybird
Rave
Ravening
Raving
Reaction
Reactive depression
Really gone
Retardation (retarded, retard)
Retardo
Rocks in his head
Room for rent
Round the bend
Ruined
Rum-dum (Rum-dumb)
Rummy
Run amuck
Running amok

S

Sadism
Sado-masochism
Sap
Sapphism
Sappy
Satanism
Satyriasis
Scattered
Scatterbrain
Schizo
Schizo-affective disorder
Schizoid
Schizophrenia
Schizothymia
Schizy

Scramblebrains

Scrambled

Scrambled egg

Scra-rewy

Screaming meemies

Screwball

Screwbally

Screw loose

Screwed

Screwed up

Screwy

Screwy skirt

Seasonal affective disorder

Seasonal depression

Self-abuse (masturbation, onanism)

Self-deceit

Self-destruction *See also*, masochism, suicide

Semantic-pragmatic deficit disorder

Senility

Senseless

Sex abuse

Sex criminal

Sex maniac

Sex offender

Sexaholic

Sexual abuse; Victim of sexual abuse

Sexual addiction

Sexual frigidity

Sexual impotence

Sexual inversion (homosexuality)

Sexual perversion

Sexual psychopath

Sexual voyeurism

S-H-A-F-T syndrome

Shallow-brain

Shallow-minded

Shambles (as in, He is a shambles;
   his life is a shambles)

Shatterbrain

Shatterpated

Shit for brains

Shit-faced

Shit-head

Short-witted

Shot

Should have his head examined

Shrink bait

Sick (sick in the head)

Sicko

Silly

Silly as a coot

Silly-head

Simple

Simple Jack

Simple-Minded

Simple Simon

The simples

Sing the blues

Skee-rewy

Slate loose

Slightly crazy

Slip a cog

The slippery slope

Slough of despond

Slug

Slow

Smash up

Smashed

Snap one's cap

Snozzlewobbes

Sociopath

Sociopathic

Sociopathy

Softhead

Soldier's heart

Sop

Space face

Space cadet

Spaced-out

Spacy

Speed freak

Split personality

Spooky

Spoony
Spouse abuse
Spring a leak (in the think tank)
Sprung
Squirrel food
Squirrels in the nut
Squirrely
Stir-bug
Stir-crazy
Stir-nut
Stir-wacky
Stolid
Stove in
Strange (e.g., a little strange)
Stress disorder
Stressed
Stuck in neutral
Stultified
Stultiloquence (foolish talk or babble)
Stupid
Stupor
Substance abuse
Substance dependence
Suicide
A suitcase without a handle
Syndrome
Syringobrainia

T

Tabacism
Tabacosis
Tachyphrenia
Take leave of one's senses
Talking ragtime
Talks nonsense
Talks senseless
Tarantism
Tards (for Re-tards)
Teaism
Teched (tetched)

Teched in the head
Thick
Thick-sculled
Tile loose
Tilt at windmills
Tobacco abuse
Tobacco dependence
Tobaccoism
Tockay
Tom Noddy
Tomfool
Too few dots on his dice
Took leave of his senses
Touch bottom
Touched
Toxic delirium
Toxic psychosis
Train doesn't stop at all the stations
Transference neurosis
Transsexualism
Transvestism
Transvestitism
Traumatic neurosis
Tribadism
Trifler
Troubled
Turkey
Turned into the wrong station
Twirly
Twisted
Twit

U

Ulcers in the brain
Unbalanced
Uncontrolled
Undifferentiated
Undone
Unhinged
Unnoodled

Unpredictable
Unreasonableness
Unsettled
Unsoundness (e.g., unsound mind)
Unteachable
Up (e.g., he is up)
Up the flue
Up the pole
Up the pole and halfway around the
    flag
Upper story is unfurnished
Uptight
Uranianism (homosexuality)
Uranism
Urningism (male homosexuality)

V

Vacancy of mind
Vacant
Vacant attic
Valetudinarianism (a condition of
    poor health)
Vasomotor neurosis
Vasoregulatory asthenia
Vegetable
Visionary
Voom-Voom
Voyeurism

W

Wack
Wacko
Wacked out
Wacky
Wacky twerp
Walking soap opera
Walking worried
Walking wounded
Wandering
Wanting

Warped
Wastoid
Water topside
Waterhead
Way out
Weak in the upper story
Wearied
Weetless
Weird
Weirded out
Weirdo
Whacked
Whacky
Wheels in the head
Wicky-wacky
Wigged out
Wires are crossed
Wiseacre
Who let him out?
Wife abuse
Will-o'-the-wisp
Wise men of Gotham
Without rhyme or reason
Witless (e.g., Half-wit; nit-wit)
Women who love too much syn-
    drome
Woobles
Woody
Wooky
World-weary
Worried
Wrapped a little loose (Not too well
    wrapped)
Wrapped too loosely
Wreck (as in, He is a wreck; his life
    is a wreck)
Wrong in the nut
Wrong in the upper story

Y

Yarmouth

Z

Zany

Zoanthropy (a form of insanity or mental disorder in which the sufferer imagines that he is an animal)

Zombie

Zoned out

Zonked

Zonked out

Zonkers

Zoopsia (a form of hallucination in which the sufferer imagines he sees animals)

Zooscopy (zoopsia)

Synonyms for Mental Hospital

> *I don't regard you as a doctor. You call this a*
> *hospital, I call it a prison. . . . So now, let's get*
> *everything straight. I am your prisoner, you are*
> *my jailer, and there isn't going to be any nonsense*
> *about my health or my relations, or about exami-*
> *nation and treatment.*
>
> —Valeriy Tarsis, *Ward* 7

As I noted earlier, a slang term may uplift (euphemism) or downcast (dysphemism). Euphemisms often become the officially correct and socially polite terms and phrases for rude or vulgar acts or things, especially body parts and sexual acts. Mencken catalogued both kinds with equal enthusiasm. Among the psychiatric "uplifters" he mentioned the following: "In the lunatic asylums (now *state hospitals* or *mental hospitals* or *psychiatric institutes*) a guard is an *attendant*, a violent patient is *assaultive*, and one whose aberration is not all-out is *maladjusted*."[16] British society was even more defensive about psychiatry than American, judging by this quaint example Mencken cites. The sentence "A *nut factory*, eh?" in a 1929 American film, had to be translated for the English cinema industry into "A *madhouse, eh*?"[17]

A personal reminiscence illustrates the persistent pressure to rename the buildings formerly called insane asylums or madhouses, but actually used to store unwanted persons. Because the ugly truth of institutional psychiatry relentlessly contradicts the sanitized names we give to such storage bins, the pressure for fresh euphemism soon builds up again. In 1956, when I moved to Syracuse, New York, the name of the local state mental hospital was the Syracuse Psychopathic Hospital. Within a year, it was renamed the Syracuse Psychiatric Center. Less than ten years later, it was renamed again, the Hutchings Psychiatric Center (after Richard Hutchings, a former commissioner of mental hygiene in New York and clinical professor of psychiatry at what was then the Syracuse University School of Medicine). Today, it is usually called simply Hutchings, without any reference to psychiatry or the state.

Adult home	Boobyhatch
Asylum	Brain sanatorium
Balm Beach	Buggery
Bathhouse	Bughouse

Clinic
Community mental health center
Community psychiatric center
Crackpothouse
Crazy house
Daffysylum
Fit House
Foolish factory
Group home
Home of the mentally bankrupt
Home of twisted nuts
Hospital for the insane (e.g., for the criminally insane)
House of cracked wits or nuts
Idiotarium
Insane asylum
Insane hospital
Loony bin
Lunatic asylum
Luniversity
Madhouse
Mental clinic
Mental health center
Mental health clinic
Mental home
Mental hospital
Mental institution
Mental rehabilitation center
Mental ward

Napoleon's Castle
Ninniversity
Nursing home
Nut Alley
Nut College
Nut Factory
Nut Farm
Nut Foundry
Nuthatch
Nut hoosegow
Nut House
Nut ward
Nuttery
Psychiatric center
Psychiatric hospital
Psychiatric institution
Psychiatric unit
Psychopathic hospital
Psychopathic ward
Residential treatment center
Rest home
Squirrel cage
Squirrel pen
Squirrel ranch
State hospital
State institution
State school
Transitional living center
VA (short for psychiatric unit of VA hospital)

4

Dictionaries of Drunkenness

*If I had a thousand sons, The first principle I
would teach them Should be to foreswear thin po-
tations, And to addict themselves to sack.*
—Shakespeare, *Second Part
of King Henry the Fourth*

Since the earliest recorded times, alcoholic beverages, the circumstances in which they are consumed, and the consequences of consuming
them have interested people nearly everywhere, but perhaps no group
more than the English-speaking people, especially Americans. Preoccupation with alcohol—as beverage, relaxant, tonic, stimulant, anesthetic,
drug, temptation, vice, article of commerce, taboo, social problem, and
illness—is reflected in the plethora of English words, both technical and
colloquial, for drunkenness. Indeed, the first list of American colloqui-
alisms on any subject was Benjamin Franklin's catalogue of synonyms
for drunkenness, *The Drinkers Dictionary*, published in 1737.

The effect of Prohibition on American English illustrates how obsession with an activity, especially if it is simultaneously prohibited by law
and promoted by custom, stimulates the production of fresh slang terms.
Because the English language and Prohibition were the two subjects
closest to Mencken's heart, it is not surprising that he had a good deal to
say about the relationship between them. He wrote:

> Prohibition increased enormously the number of American boozers, both relatively and
> absolutely, and made the whole nation booze-conscious, and as a result its everyday speech
> was peppered with terms having to do with the traffic in strong drink, *e.g.*, *bootlegger*,
> *bathtub-gin*, *rum-runner*, *bone-dry*, *needle-beer*, and *jake* (Jamaica ginger).[1]

Mencken revels in the rain forest of terms that sprung up from the soil
of American English fertilized with the manure of Prohibition. For
example, he notes that the term *saloon* became so tainted by anti-alcohol

propaganda that, after Prohibition was repealed, the name never resumed its former place in our language. "So far as I know," wrote Mencken in 1961, "there is not a single undisguised *saloon* in the United States today. They are *taverns*, *cocktail-lounges*, *taprooms*, *beer-stubes*, or the like. Some are even called *bars*, *lounge-bars* or *cocktail-bars*, but *saloon* seems to be definitely out."[2] The same sort of linguistic revisionism is at work in the transformation of *Negro* into *colored*, *black*, and *African-American*; of *insane* into *manic-depressive* and *bipolar*; and of *state hospital* into *psychiatric center*.

Other connoisseurs of language beside Mencken have remarked on the effects of Prohibition on the American language, among them Edmund Wilson. His "Lexicon of Prohibition," published in 1927, is also reprinted below.

Benjamin Franklin's "The Drinkers Dictionary"

Were I to commence my administration again, . . .
the first question I would ask respecting a candi-
date would be, "Does he use ardent spirits?"
—Thomas Jefferson

"The Drinkers Dictionary" was originally published anonymously, in the *Pennsylvania Gazette*, in January 1737.[3] It consisted of an alphabetical arrangement of more than two hundred and twenty-five synonyms or synonymous phrases denoting drunkenness, and was introduced by a quotation from Franklin's *Poor Richard's Almanack*.

Franklin scholars are unanimous in their judgment that "The Dictionary" was compiled by Benjamin Franklin.[4] In 1722, when Franklin was only sixteen, he had already collected nineteen terms signifying drunkenness. Fifteen of them appear, with slight changes, in "The Drinkers Dictionary."[5] Cedric Larson, who cites original sources from the rare books collection of the Library of Congress, emphasizes that the fact that the *Gazette* was owned in part by Franklin, together with other convincing evidence, leaves little doubt that the "Dictionary" was compiled by Franklin himself. Franklin was, indeed, much concerned with the problem we now call alcoholism. For example, he devoted almost the entire issue of the *Pennsylvania Gazette* of 22 July 1736 to a report on the ravages of drunkenness in England, "as a warning to the colonists."[6]

Nevertheless, Franklin was anything but a critic of drinking. In an undated letter, he sings the praises of wine, while poking fun, gently but wisely, at water drinkers:

In vino veritas, says the sage, *truth in wine.* Before Noah, therefore, men, having nothing but Water to drink, could not find out the Truth. Thus, they erred, they became dreadfully Wicked, and they were fittingly exterminated by the Water they liked to drink.

Goodman Noah, having seen that all his Contemporaries had perished by this unwholesome drink, took an aversion to it, and God, to quench his thirst, created the Grape, and revealed the art of making Wine from it. By means of this LIQUOR he discovered many and many a Truth; and since this time, the word *Divine* has been used, originally meaning *Divination by Wine.* . . . Thus, from that time, all excellent things, even Gods, have been called *divine* or *divinities.*[7]

A fanatic for moderation, Franklin was as sure that drunkenness was a vice as we, fanatics for medicine, are that it is a disease.[8] With his keen ear for language, he noted, moreover, that drunkenness was unlike most other vices, which "always endeavour to assume the Appearance of Virtue: Thus Covetousness calls itself *Prudence*; *Prodigality* would be thought of as *Generosity;* and so of others."[9] Not so with intemperate drinking:

> But DRUNKENNESS is a very unfortunate Vice in this respect. It bears no kind of Similitude with any sort of Virtue, from which it might possibly borrow a Name; and is therefore reduc'd to the wretched Necessity of being express'd by distant round-about Phrases, and of perpetually varying those Phrases, as often as they come to be well understood to signify plainly that A MAN IS DRUNK.[10]

In 1737, Franklin would not have dreamed that he would become one of the founders of a great new country, whose people would collectively decide to ban their favorite beverage only to defy the prohibition, and who would then construct a complex, pseudomedical vocabulary for the sole purpose of denying that there is anything at all *plain* about drinking or being a drunkard.[11]

The Drinker's Dictionary[12]

Nothing more like a Fool than a drunken Man.
—Poor Richard

A

He is Addled,
He's casting up his Accounts,
He's Afflicted,
He's in his Airs.

B

He's Biggy,
  Bewitch'd,
  Block and Block,
  Boozy,
  Bowz'd,
  Been at Barbadoes,
  Piss'd in the Brook,
  Drunk as a Wheel-Barrow,
  Burdock'd,
  Buskey,
  Buzzey,
Has stole a Manchet out of the
  Brewer's Basket,
His Head is full of Bees,
Has been in the Bibbing Plot,
Has drank more than he has bled,
He's Bungey,
As Drunk as a Beggar,
He sees the Bears,
He's kiss'd black Betty,
He's had a Thump over the Head
  with Sampson's Jawbone,
He's Bridgey.

C

He's Cat,
  Cagrin'd,
  Capable,

Cramp'd,
Cherubimical,
Cherry Merry,
Wamble Crop'd,
Crack'd,
Concern'd,
Half Way to Concord,
Has taken a Chirriping Glass,
  Got Corns in his Head,
  A Cup too much,
  Coguy,
  Copey,
He's heat his Copper,
He's Crocus,
  Catch'd,
He cuts his Capers,
He's been in the Cellar,
He's in his Cups,
  Non Compos,
  Cock'd,
  Curv'd,
  Cut,
  Chipper,
  Chickery,
  Loaded his Cart,
He's been too free with the Creature,
Sir Richard has taken off his Con-
  sidering Cap,
He's Chap-fallen.

D

He's Disguiz'd,
He's got a Dish,
  Kill'd his Dog,
  Took his Drops,
It is a Dark Day with him,
He's a Dead Man,

Has Dipp'd his Bill,
He's Dagg'd,
He's seen the Devil.

E

He's Prince Eugene,
   Enter'd,
   Wet both Eyes,
   Cock Ey'd,
   Got the Pole Evil,
   Got a brass Eye,
   Made an Example,
He's eat a Toad & Half for Break-
   fast,
   In his Element.

F

He's Fishey,
   Fox'd,
   Fuddled,
   Sore Footed,
   Frozen,
   Well in for't,
   Owes no Man a Farthing,
   Fears no Man,
   Crump Footed,
   Been to France,
   Flush'd,
   Froze his Mouth,
   Fetter'd,
   Been to a Funeral,
   His Flag is out,
   Fuzl'd,
   Spoke with his Friend,
   Been at an Indian Feast.

G

He's Glad,
   Groatable,
   Gold-headed,

Glaiz'd,
Generous,
Booz'e the Gage,
As Dizzy as a Goose,
Been before George,
Got the Gout,
Had a Kick in the Guts,
Been with Sir John Goa,
Been at Geneva,
Globular,
Got the Glanders.

H

Half and Half,
Hardy,
Top Heavy,
Got by the Head,
Hiddey,
Got on his little Hat,
Hammerish,
Loose in the Hilts,
Knows not the way Home,
Got the Hornson,
Haunted with Evil Spirits,
Has taken Hippocrates grand Elixir.

I

He's Intoxicated,
   Jolly,
   Jagg'd,
   Jambled,
   Going to Jerusalem,
   Jocular,
   Been to Jerico,
   Juicy.

K

He's a King,
   Clips the King's English,
   Seen the French King,

The King is his Cousin,
Got Kib'd Heels,
Knapt,
Het his Kettle,

L

He's in Liquor,
Lordly,
He makes Indentures with his
Leggs,
Well to live,
Light,
Lappy,
Limber.

M

He sees two Moons,
Merry,
Middling,
Moon-ey'd,
Muddled,
Seen a Flock of Moons,
Maudlin,
Mountous,
Muddy
Rais'd his Monuments,
Mellow.

N

He's eat the Cocoa Nut,
Nimptopsical,
Got the Night Mare.

O

He's Oil'd,
Eat Opium,
Smelt of an Onion,

Oxycrocium,
Overset.

P

He drank till he gave up his Half-
Penny,
Pidgeon Ey'd,
Pungey,
Priddy,
As good conditioned as a Puppy,
Has scalt his Head Pan,
Been among the Philistines,
In his Prosperity,
He's been among the Philippians,
He's contending with Pharaoh,
Wasted his Paunch,
He's Polite,
Eat a Pudding Bagg.

Q

He's Quarrelsome.

R

He's Rocky,
Raddled,
Rich,
Religious,
Lost his Rudder,
Ragged,
Rais'd,
Been too free with Sir Richard,
Like a Rat in Trouble.

S

He's Stitch'd,
Seafaring,
In the Sudds,

Strong,
Been in the Sun.
As drunk as David's Sow,
Swampt,
His Skin is full,
He's Steady,
He's Stiff,
He's burnt his Shoulder,
He's got his Top Gallant Sails out,
    Seen the yellow Star,
    As Stiff as a Ring-bolt,
    Half Seas over,
    His Shoe pinches him,
    Staggerish,
    It is Star-light with him,
He carries too much Sail,
Stew'd,
Stubb'd,
Soak'd,
Soft,
Been too free with Sir John
    Strawberry,
He's right before the Wind with all
    his Studding Sails out,
Has Sold his Senses.

T

He's Top'd,
    Tongue-ty'd,

Tann'd,
Tipium Grove,
Double Tongu'd,
Topsy Turvey,
Tipsey,
Has Swallow'd a Tavern Token,
He's Thaw'd,
He's in a Trance,
He's Trammel'd.

V

He makes Virginia Fence,
    Valiant,
    Got the Indian Vapours.

W

The Malt is above the Water,
He's Wise,
He's Wet,
He's been to the Salt Water,
He's Water-soaken,
He's very Weary,
    Out of the Way.

Edmund Wilson's "The Lexicon of Prohibition"[13]

*Mississippi will drink wet and vote dry so long as
any citizen can stagger to the polls.*
—Will Rogers

I reprint below the complete text of Wilson's short piece, save for his
closing remarks, which run to about two hundred fifty words. The gist
of his remarks is that "the social vocabulary of drinking, as exemplified
by this list, seems to have become especially rich: one gets the impression
that more nuances are nowadays discriminated than was the case before
Prohibition."[14]

The Lexicon of Prohibition

The following is a partial list of words denoting drunkenness now in
common use in the United States. They have been arranged, as far as
possible, in order of the degrees of intensity of the conditions which they
represent, beginning with the mildest stages and progressing to the more
disastrous.

lit
squiffy
oiled
lubricated
owled
edged
jingled
piffed
piped
sloppy
woozy
happy
half-screwed
half-cocked
half-shot
half seas over
fried

stewed
boiled
zozzled
sprung
scrooched
jazzed
jagged
canned
corked
corned
potted
hooted
slopped
tanked
stinko
blind
stiff

under the table
tight
full
wet
high
horseback
liquored
pickled
ginned
shicker (Yiddish)
spifflicated
primed
organized
featured
pie-eyed
cock-eyed
wall-eyed
glassy-eyed
bleary-eyed
hoary-eyed
over the Bay
four sheets in the wind
crocked
loaded
leaping
screeching
lathered
plastered
soused
bloated
polluted
saturated
full as a tick
loaded for bear
loaded to the muzzle
loaded to the plimsoll mark

wapsed down
paralyzed
ossified
out like a light
passed out cold
embalmed
buried
blotto
lit up like the sky
lit up like the Commonwealth
lit up like a Christmas tree
lit up like a store window
lit up like a church
fried to the hat
slopped to the ears
stewed to the gills
boiled as an owl
to have a bun on
to have a slant on
to have a skate on
to have a snootful
to have a skinful
to draw a blank
to pull a shut-eye
to pull a Daniel Boone
to have a rubber drink
to have a hangover
to have a head
to have the jumps
to have the shakes
to have the zings
to have the heeby-jeebies
to have the screaming-meemies
to have the whoops and jingles
to burn with a low blue flame

Contemporary Dictionary of Drunkenness[15]

Candy is dandy, But liquor is quicker.
—Ogden Nash

A

Addict
Alcohol abuse
Alcohol addicted
Alcohol dependent
Alcoholic
Alkied
All geezed up
All mops and brooms
Aped
As stiff as a ring bolt

B

Back teeth afloat
Balmy
Bamboozled
Barfly
Basted
Battered
Bay, over the
Been to Barbados
Befuddled
Behind the cork
Belt the grape
Bend the elbow
Bent
Biggy
Blacked out
Black-out (gray-out)
Bleary-eyed
Blind

Blinded
Blink, on the
Bloated
Blotto
Blown
Blown up
Blue
Blue around the gills
Blue-eyed
Boiled
Boozed
Boozed up
Boozer
Boozy
Bottled
Bowzed
Bowzered
Brandy Nan
Beezy
Brick in one's hat
Bridgey
Bruised
Bungey
Bunned
Buried
Burn with a low blue flame
Buzzed
Buzzey

C

Caged
Canned

Canned up
Carry a (heavy) load
Cat
Chemically dependent
Cherry-merry
Cherubimical
Chug-a-lug
Clobbered
Cocked
Cockeyed
Comfortable
Cooked
Corked
Corned
Crocked
Cronk
Crump
Crumped
Crumped out
Cuckooed
Cut

D

Dagged
Damaged
D and D
Dead to the world
Decks awash
Ding-swizzled
Dipped his bill
Discouraged
Disguised
Down the hatch
Draw a blank
Drenched
Drink like a fish
Drug dependent
Drunk
Drunk as a bartender on his night off
Drunk as a beesom

Drunk as a beggar
Drunk as a boiled owl
Drunk as a fiddler
Drunk as a fiddler's bitch
Drunk as a fish
Drunk as a goat
Drunk as a goose
Drunk as a horse-fly
Drunk as a lord
Drunk as a mouse
Drunk as a pig
Drunk as a piper all day long
Drunk as a Plymouth fiddler
Drunk as a rat
Drunk as a skunk
Drunk as a stewed owl
Drunk as a swine
Drunk as a tinker
Drunk as a wheel-barrow
Drunk as an ape
Drunk as an emperor
Drunk as David's sow (Swift)
Drunk as Davy's sow
Drunk as hogs
Drunk as owls
Drunk as the Baltic sea
Drunk as the devil

E

Edged
Elevated
Embalmed
Ethanol abuse

F

Faint
Feel as if a cat has kittened in one's
    mouth
Feel good

Feel no pain
Fired up
Fish-eyed
Fishy
Fishy about the gills
Floating
Flooey
Fogmatic
Folded
Four sheets to (in) the wind
Foxed
Fractured
Frazzled
Fresh
Fried
Fried up
Fucked up
Fuddled
Full
Full as an egg
Full as a tick
Fuzzled
Fuzzy

G

Gaged
Gassed
Gay
Gayed
Geared up
Geezed
Giggle water
Ginned
Ginned up
Glassy
Glassy eyed
Glaized
Glazed
Glowed
Glued

Gold-headed
Gone
Got a brass eye
Gray-out (black-out)
Greased
Grogged
Guyed out
Guzzled

H

Half-cocked
Half-corned
Half-crocked
Half-screwed
Half seas over
Half shaved
Half-shot
Half-slewed
Half-snapped
Half-sprung
Half-stewed
Half the bay over
Half the bay under
Half under
Hammered Hang one on
Happy
Has bet his kettle
Has his flag out
Have a bag on
Have a bun on
Have a can on
Have a glow on
Have a jag on
Have a package on
Have a snoot full
Have an edge on
Have one for the worms
Have one's gage up
Have one's pots on
Have the sun in one's eyes

Heeled
Here's mud in your eye
High
High as a kite
Higher than a kite
High lonesome
Hipped
Hoary-eyed
Hooted
Hot
How come ye so

I

Illuminated
In bed with one's boots on
In good humor
In his airs
In one's cups
In the altitudes
In the bag
In the gutter
In very good humor
Inebriated
Intoxicated

J

Jagged
Jammed
Jazzed
Jingled
John Barleycorn
Jolly
Jug-bitten
Jugged
Jug-steamed
Juiced
Juiced up

K

Killed
Kited
Knocked for a loop
Knocked out

L

Laid out
Lappy
Lathered
Like an owl in an ivy bush
Limber
Limp
Lined
Liquored
Liquored up
Lit
Lit to the gills
Lit to the guards
Lit up
Lit up like a Christmas tree (Main
    Street, Times Square, Broadway,
    a store window, a church, etc.)
Loaded
Loaded for bear
Loaded to the gills (the muzzle, the
    plimsoll mark, etc.)
Looped
Looped-legged
Loopy
Loose in the hilt
Lordly
Lubricated
Lush
Lushed
Lushed up

M

Malt above the meal
Mellow
Melted
Merry
Mokus
Moon-eyed
Mulled
Mulled up

N

Nimptopsical

O

Oiled
On the lee lurch
On the sauce
On the shikker
One for the road
One over the eight
On the sauce
Organized
Orie-eyed
Ossified
Out like a light
Out of the way
Out on the roof
Overboard
Overset
Owly-eyed

P

Packaged
Paralyzed
Parboiled
Parson Palmer
Petrified
Pickled

Pie-eyed
Piffed
Pifficated
Piffled
Pifflicated
Pigeon-eyed
Pilfered
Pinked
Piped
Pixilated
Plastered
Plonked
Polished up
Polluted
Potted
Potted up
Potty
Preserved
Primed
Pruned
Put to bed with a shovel

Q

Queer in the attic

R

Raddled
Raunchy
Ready
Rigid
Rileyed
Ripe
Rocky
Rosy
Rum-dum
Rush the growler

S

Salted down
Sap-happy

Sapped saturated
Sawed
Scraunched
Screaming
Screeching
Screwed
Scronched
Seafaring in the suds
Seen the devil
Sent
Set-up
Sewed up
Shaved
Shellacked
Shikker
Shikkered
Shined
Shit-faced
Shoot the cat
Shot
Shot in the neck
Skunked
Slewed
Slopped
Slopped over
Sloppy
Sloshed
Slugged
Smash the teapot
Smashed
Smoked
Snapped
Snokered
Snookered
Snozzled
Snubbed
Snuffy
Soaked
Soshed
Soused
Soused to the gills
Sozzled

Spiffed
Spifflicated
Splice the main brace
Sprung
Squiffed
Squiffy
Staggering
Staggering drunk
Stewed
Stewed to the gills
Stewed up
Sticked
Stiff
Stiff as a ring bolt
Stinking
Stinkarooed
Stinko
Stitched
Stone blind
Stoned
Striped
Stunned
Substance abuse
Suck the monkey
Swacked
Swazzled
Swiped
Swizzeld
Swozzled

T

Tangle-footed
Tangle-legged
Tanked
Tanked up
Tap the admiral
Teed up
Three sheets in the wind
Tiddly
Tie one on
Tight

Tight as a tick
Tipped
Tippy
Tipsey
Tipsy
Top-heavy
Troll the bowl
Tuned
Turned on

U

Under the table
Under the weather
Unsteady
Up to the gills

V

Vulcanized

W

Walk the chalk

Wall-eyed
Wapsed down
Weak jointed
Wear the barley cap
Well oiled
Wet
Wet one's whistle
Whipped
Whipsey
Whooshed
Wilted
Wine of ape
Wing-heavy
Wooden leg (he has a ...)
Woofled
Woozy

Z

Zig-Zag
Zonked out
Zonkered

II

METAPHORIC MALADY, MORAL RESPONSIBILITY, AND PSYCHIATRY

5

The Religion Called "Psychiatry"

*Well then, maybe it would be worth mentioning
the three periods of history. When man believed
that happiness was dependent upon God, he
killed for religious reasons. When he believed
that happiness was dependent upon the form of
government, he killed for political reasons. . . .
After dreams that were too long, true nightmares.
. . . we arrived at the present period of history.
Man woke up, discovered that which we always
knew, that happiness is dependent upon health,
and began to kill for therapeutic reasons. . . . It is
medicine that has come to replace both religion
and politics in our time.*

—Adolfo Bioy Casares,
"Plans for an Escape to Carmelo"

The most obvious thing about psychiatry has always seemed to me to
be the fact that psychiatrists have the power to deprive their patients of
liberty; in other words, that a group of physicians is legally and medically
authorized to incarcerate persons who have been neither charged with,
nor convicted of, a crime. It thus follows, as night follows day, that
commitment is an act of blatant coercion, regardless of how it might be
justified. Of course, in real life, social customs and their moral justifications go hand in hand; thus, it is axiomatic that all legal coercions are
"justified." What requires attention, then, is the various ways in which
people have justified coercion in the past, and justify it today.

For millennia, people have viewed theological arguments as true, and
hence as valid justifications for coercing persons who have not deprived
anyone of life, liberty, or property. Many people—for example, millions
of Muslims who believe Salman Rushdie deserves to be killed—still
share that view and consider it a lofty vision. We call such persons

religious fanatics, a diagnosis that makes us feel smug and superior to them. But shouldn't we judge ourselves by similar criteria—that is, by asking: What argument do we regard as at once so important and so true that its rejection justifies coercing persons who have not deprived anyone of life, liberty, or property? The answer is obvious: We seek truth in what Science "tells us," much as our forebears sought truth in what God "told them." We believe in mental illness and psychiatric treatment, much as our forebears believed in possession and exorcism. And we use the ideas of mental illness and psychiatric treatment to justify punishing innocent persons, just as our forebears used the ideas of possession and exorcism to do so.

It is important to keep in mind that the practice of psychiatry, as we now know it, began a little over three hundred years ago with the confining of mad persons in insane asylums. How was this procedure justified? By the idea, unknown and undreamt of before the seventeenth century, that insanity is unreason, and that, in the asylum, unreason could be turned back into reason and hence sanity. The prospect of future sanity thus served to justify the practice of present segregation. In the course of the next three centuries, justifying coercion by therapy became as dear to the heart of modern secular man as justifying coercion by theology had ever been to the heart of medieval man.

Let us now consider some specific parallels between religion and psychiatry, by focusing on the ideas and acts most abhorred by each of these systems of belief and social control. The core act of deviance in religion is blasphemy or heresy; in psychiatry, it is delusion or psychosis.

To appreciate the similarities between blasphemy and psychosis, all we need to do is set them in the context of freedom of speech. Commentators on First Amendment freedoms are fond of citing Justice Oliver Wendell Holmes's following phrase to illustrate what this principle ought to mean. He wrote: "The principle of the Constitution that most imperatively calls for our attachment is 'not free thought for those who agree with us but freedom for the thought that we hate.'"[1] In this light, consider these two typical utterances:

"Jesus is not the son of God, but the son of man."
"I am Jesus and must help men to see the Truth."

The person who uttered the first statement—denying the divinity of Jesus—was considered to be a blasphemer in medieval Catholic countries. The person who utters the second statement—denying reality—is considered to be psychotic in modern, Western countries. It would be uncritical intellectual acquiescence to dismiss such cases as instances of religious or psychiatric "abuse." On the contrary, they are typical examples of religious and psychiatric justifications for social control —of which, if we (later) disapprove, we call "persecution." An unbridgeable gulf separates such ideologies of intolerant conceit from love of peace and respect for human diversity. The latter posture—characterized by modesty and self-restraint—is well illustrated in one of Thomas Jefferson's letters, written in 1808, to his grandson, Thomas Jefferson Randolph:

> When I hear another express an opinion, which is not mine, I say to myself, he has a right to his opinion, as I to mine, why should I question it? His error does me no injury; and shall I become a Don Quixote, to bring all men by force of argument to one opinion? If a fact be misstated, it is probable that he is gratified by a belief of it, and I have no right to deprive him of the gratification. If he wants information, he will ask it, and then I will give it in measured terms; but if he still believes his own story, and shows a desire to dispute the facts with me, I hear him and say nothing. It is his affair, not mine, if he prefers error.[2]

We are ready now to view psychotherapy as religion. Because the term *psychotherapy* has become vague and all-encompassing, I shall direct my attention to the paradigmatic psychotherapeutic enterprise of psychoanalysis.

Freud was anxious to define what he did as scientific, and to deny that it had anything to do with religion. Why? Briefly put, because for Freud *religion* was a bad word—synonymous with *illusion, irrationality,* and *intolerance*; and *science* was a good word—synonymous with *truth, tolerance,* and *therapy*. For me, and for many people today, this is a facile and foolish generalization. In fact, *religion* may be either a good or a bad word—signifying weakness or strength, irrationality or inspiration, intolerance or courage; *science,* too, may be a good or a bad word—denoting truth or error, tolerance or authoritarianism, therapy or torture.[3] As mere abstractions, religion and science are simply blank checks; in actuality, each is what we, fallible and fallen human beings, make of them. In short, I regard neither religion nor science as all good or all bad; and I classify psychoanalysis as a religion rather than as a science neither to condemn it nor to praise it, but rather to identify it correctly—as a quasi-religious (ideological) system and practice, in competition with other such systems and practices. Whether, as a practical matter, we consider psychoanalysis to be good or bad will depend on the nature of the relationship between therapist and patient, and on our personal judgment of it.[4]

Actually, the view that psychoanalytic treatment is a type of religious counseling was suggested by Freud himself. He wrote:

> The words, "secular pastoral worker," might well serve as a general formula for describing the function of the analyst. . . . we do not seek to bring [the patient] relief by receiving him into the catholic, protestant, or socialist community. We seek rather to enrich him from his own internal sources... Such activity as this is pastoral work in the best sense of the word.[5]

Unfortunately, this statement is inconsistent with Freud's unqualified rejection of the value of religion—especially since he knew perfectly well that, prior to the twentieth century, people looked to religion for help with their problems in living. Today, people look to psychotherapy for it. We fool ourselves if we ignore the competition and conflict between these two approaches; and we imperil ourselves if we declare the psychotherapeutic approach scientific and therefore legitimate, and the religious approach unscientific and therefore illegitimate.

In 1886, when Freud was thirty years old, he opened his office in Vienna as a specialist in neurology. The German word for such a specialist was *Nervenarzt*, literally, "nerve doctor." His counterpart in English-speaking countries was called a specialist in "diseases of the nervous system" or in "nervous diseases." Patients came to Freud for the diagnosis and treatment of "nervous diseases"—whatever that term meant to them, their relatives, and their doctors; and the specialist in such diseases had to offer the patients something to justify his intervention as medical, and for charging them. From an economic point of view, Freud's model, Jean-Martin Charcot, the famous French neurologist and neuropathologist —and other hospital-based specialists in nervous diseases— had it much easier. They worked for, and received a salary from, a hospital or state bureaucracy. Moreover, their patients were indigent persons housed in institutions, whom the doctors, who were not their agents, had no incentive to please. On the contrary, these early alienists, neurologists, and neuropathologists could simply study their patients, as long as they were alive, as so many "interesting cases"— and, after they died, as cadavers who were "materials for dissection." Obviously, patients who had money and occupied a higher social position than their physicians could not be so easily used and abused. Moreover, these private patients suffering from "neuroses" had nothing demonstrably wrong with them—and usually outlived their physicians. Faced with such a customer, the privately practicing physician had to offer something that society legitimized as a treatment and the patient considered worth paying for. Since, as a rule, there was no treatment for what ailed patients (the more so if their diseases were metaphoric), the physician had to pretend that he could do something to help, and had to call whatever he did a "treatment." The complementary pretendings of patient and psychiatrist thus originated from the cultural-social situation in which psychoanalysis and modern psychotherapy were born and developed.

Throughout his long professional life, Freud maintained that his patients suffered from a class of diseases called "neuroses," and that he treated them with a special method he called "psychoanalysis." Probably he believed all this. But what is a neurosis? What did Freud think "it" was?

Our present ideas about the nature of mental disorders are badly confused. In Freud's day, people's ideas on this subject were even more confused. Today's psychiatrists want to know what sorts of diseases neurotic disorders *are*. In Freud's day, they wanted to know what *caused* them. After all, the term *neurosis* presupposes that "it" is a disease of neurones or nerves. It is not surprising that, despite the differences between the roles of physician and psychoanalyst, Freud insisted, especially when it suited his purposes, that psychoanalysis was simply a type of medical treatment. "The theory of the neuroses," he declared in 1917, "is a chapter in medicine, like any other."[6] Fifteen years later, he wrote: "Psychoanalysis is really a treatment like others," and then added: "and here I should like to add that I do not think our cures can compete with those of Lourdes."[7]

But if psychoanalysis is a medical treatment, why did Freud compare it to the cures offered at Lourdes? Because, in fact, psychoanalysis is more like a ceremonial "treatment." Unlike the physician or surgeon who typically does something *to* the patient, the analyst only communicates *with* him. Through such acts of carefully structured listening and speaking, the analyst engages in ministerial rather than medical work. Moreover, Freud knew—and acknowledged—that his role as therapist consisted of listening and talking *only*. "My practice," he wrote to his friend Wilhelm Fliess, in 1888, "is not very considerable, [but] has recently benefitted somewhat because of the name of Charcot. The carriage is expensive, and visiting, and *talking people into and out of things, which is what my work consists of,* robs me of the best time for work."[8] In short, the hysteric felt compelled to conceal her unhappiness about her sexual situation behind a veil of neurological symptoms—which she regarded, and wanted others to regard, as a bona fide illness. Similarly, Freud felt compelled to conceal his unhappiness about his work situation behind a veil of neurological symbols—which he regarded, and wanted others to regard, as a bona fide treatment.

The thesis that psychoanalysis is a religion is not new: Several of Freud's contemporary critics proposed it.[9] Indeed, the thesis is self-evident: Inasmuch as psychoanalysis deals with how we should live, it addresses the same questions religion addresses, and it prescribes and proscribes rules of conduct much as religions do.

One of the earliest and most astute critics of psychoanalysis was Karl Kraus (1874–1936), a Viennese journalist and satirist. Kraus quick recognized not only the falsehood inherent in Freud's medical claims, but also that Freud's pseudomedical idiom and ideology was fundamentally antagonistic to the basic Western values of personal freedom and responsibility. Satirizing psychoanalysis as "the disease which it claims to cure," Kraus lashed out against the psychoanalysts—whom he called "soul-suckers"—and concluded: "Despite its deceptive terminology, psychoanalysis is not a science but a religion—the faith of a generation incapable of any other."[10]

Because psychoanalysis is so closely linked to Freud's persona, and because Freud went out of his way to identify psychoanalysis as a science and himself as a scientist neutral toward religion, I shall further support my argument with quotes from Freud's writings as well as with examples of his personal conduct.

Freud consistently claimed that psychoanalysis is neutral toward religion. For example, in a letter to a Protestant clergyman, he wrote: "In itself psychoanalysis is neither religious nor the opposite, but an impartial instrument . . . when it is used only to free suffering people."[11] This is naively disingenuous: How can the effort "to free suffering people" be a morally impartial enterprise? From what kind of suffering was Freud offering to free people? From suffering due to sexual inhibition? From suffering due to religious oppression? And how did he propose to achieve this goal? By setting the sufferers against their own sexual codes and religious traditions?

Hiding behind the skirt of positivistic natural science, Freud methodically evaded such vexing moral questions and simply ignored the fact that—unlike physics, which deals with inanimate objects—psychoanalysis addresses the human predicament. His evasion is summed up in one of his own sentences: "In point of fact psychoanalysis is a method of research, an impartial instrument, like the infinitesimal calculus, as it were."[12] Perhaps Freud believed the absurdity that psychoanalysis is "an impartial instrument like the infinitesimal calculus." But his own words elsewhere suggest that he knew better—that, in fact, he was eager to enlist the (pseudo)science of psychoanalysis in the struggle against religion. For example, in 1901, he wrote: "One could venture to explain in this way [as psychological processes], the myths of paradise and the fall of man, of God, of good and evil, of immortality, and so on, and to transform *metaphysics* into *metapsychology*."[13]

However, what Freud pretentiously calls "metapsychology" is nothing but a subtle effort to de-ethicize the Judeo-Christian rules of conduct. Asserting that psychoanalysis has made us "recognize religious doctrines as illusions,"[14] Freud in fact proffered a new religion as if it were a new science: "My illusions are not, like religious ones, incapable of correction. . . . No, our science [psychoanalysis] is no illusion. But an illusion it would be to suppose that what science cannot give us we can get elsewhere."[15]

Freud could not have been more wrong. Actually, science can give us *only* knowledge and power (in the sense of technological control). It cannot give us many of the things we most need and want: it cannot give us love, beauty, or control over political despotism. Ironically, totalitarian politics was the great threat that stared Freud in the face throughout his whole life; yet Freud turned a persistently blind eye to it. Observing the birth and growth of the Soviet Union, he commented:

> I have no concern with an economic criticism of the communist system; I cannot enquire into whether the abolition of private property is expedient or advantageous. . . . At a time when the great nations announce that they expect salvation only from the maintenance of Christian piety, the revolution in Russia—in spite of all its disagreeable details—seems none the less like the message of a better future.[16]

Ever since the early days of psychoanalysis, many analysts proudly proclaimed that Marx's and Freud's doctrines were complementary. They were right, but not in the complimentary way they intended. The Marxist-Freudian analysts believed that communism and psychoanalysis were grand ideologies for the liberation of man; I maintain that they are exemplars of the pseudoscientific religions of our age.

Every religion offers a blueprint of the Right Way to live life. In religious systems, the Right Way is revealed by God; in scientific (scientistic) systems, by Science. The validity of Judaism, Christianity, and Islam lies in the truths that God revealed to their respective prophets. Similarly, the validity of communism lies in the truths that the allegedly scientific method of dialectical materialism revealed to its prophet, Marx; and the validity of psychoanalysis lies in the truths that the allegedly scientific method of psychoanalysis revealed to its prophet, Freud. Not by accident, both of these new religions have declared war on the old ones: Marxism views religion as an opiate, psychoanalysis, as an illusion.

Actually, unlike Copernicus and Darwin, to whom Freud liked to compare himself, the inventor of psychoanalysis made no discoveries whatever about the external world. Instead, he put forth certain rules about how we ought to speak and think about human behavior, especially conflicts between individuals and between persons and social institutions; and he succeeded in convincing many people to adopt his style of speaking and thinking about the human condition, and his recommendations for the proper ordering of human relationships. That was his achievement, and a momentous achievement it is. But it is the achievement of a religious leader that has little to do with truth, and less with science.

In this connection, it is worth noting that, in contrast to the sciences, which are not named after an individual, the world's great religions are identified precisely thus. Moses gave us the Mosaic religion, Christ gave us Christianity, Buddha gave us Buddhism, Marx gave us Marxism, and Freud gave us Freudianism. Also, as his biographers all agree, Freud was extraordinarily concerned about distinguishing his "true" teachings from the "false" teachings of his heretical disciples. Thus, to keep the Freudian faith pure, he organized a worldwide labor union of accredited analysts—the International Psychoanalytic Association.

Revealingly, Freud viewed his work as a veritable mission and called it "the cause." And, like other modern gnostic leaders, he defined himself as a liberator. From what? From what he regarded as the twin incubi of the human soul—religion and neurosis. Pitting himself explicitly against religion and offering to cure us of our need for it, he declared: "At such cost—by the forcible imposition of mental infantilism and inducing a mass-delusion—religion succeeds in saving many people from individual neuroses."[17]

Thus, Freud implied, and no doubt believed, that "neurosis" is a universal malady to which we must either submit ·or which we must overcome with the aid of psychoanalysis (only he, by means of "self analysis," could overcome it without a formal analysis). If we submit to the universal neurosis, we can choose to let religion make us sicker: By giving ourselves over to a "mass delusion," we can protect ourselves from individual neurosis. Freud mocks the common man for embracing this option. Instead, to those prepared to follow his own example of seeking the meaning of life in Psychoanalysis, he offers his (un-Christian) Science, guaranteed to save the "analyzed" from individual psychopathology (neurosis) and collective psychosis (nonpsychoanalytic religion) alike.

The ancient prophets concealed their megalomania by claiming that God spoke to them. The new prophets—Marx and Freud —conceal their megalomania by claiming that science speaks to them. But God and science are silent. However, conceited men love to speak in their names.

What has Marxist science told the Communists? It has told them, among other things, to wage war on religion. And what does Freudian science tell the psychoanalysts? The same thing. The outcomes of these wars are interesting. Because Marxist orthodoxy correctly regarded psychoanalysis as a religion, psychoanalysis was outlawed in the Soviet Union. In the United States, for exactly the opposite reason, the result has been exactly the opposite: Accepted as a bona fide science and a medical treatment, in America psychoanalysis (and the psychiatry it authenticated) flourished and, in part, replaced the theological foundations of morals and law. Moreover, because unlike the Soviet state, the American state eschews ascribing religious status to individuals or institutions that claim no such status for themselves, psychoanalysis escaped being classified as a cult. Nevertheless, psychoanalysis is a pseudomedical cult, with its secret archives in Washington, and its holy shrine in London.

In the past, priests had power. Today, psychiatrists have power. We may view such facts either as solutions or as problems. Formerly, anxious about their fate in an everlasting life in the hereafter, people relinquished their self-governance to priests—and thus gained a sense of security about their spiritual health. In the modern world, anxious about their fate here on earth, people relinquish their self-governance to doctors, especially to mind doctors—and thus gain a sense of security about their mental health. Clearly, so long as we view this sort of paternalism as a solution, we shall try to perfect its uses and reduce its so-called abuses. On the other hand, if we view such paternalism, especially exercised by a physician-agent of the state, as a problem; and if we question the high-minded pretext with which such persons justify their use power—then there is hope of our being able to limit or even abolish the use of such power.

Naturally, reformers, social activists, therapists, and other professional meddlers always claim to be using force to do good. Moreover, the justificatory image and idiom invoked usually covers both consensual and coerced relationships—which is a fatal trap for the unwary. In a free society, acts between consenting adults are permissible because they betoken the freedom of the actors, not because the actions or their consequences are necessarily beneficial: We can buy and sell cars and houses regardless of whether the transaction "benefits" anyone. The occurrence of the transaction is, itself, proof that it is "good" for at least one of the parties, and perhaps for both. Finally, in a free society, bestowing benefits cannot justify coercing the would-be beneficiary: A person cannot compel another to buy or sell, say, stocks, even if he could prove that his beneficiary would profit from the transaction.

Unlike consensual, commercial transactions, psychiatric transactions are typically nonconsensual and coercive. Why? Because, as a people, we believe in mental health and mental illness, much as our ancestors believed in God and Satan. The struggle for God and against Satan was the grand legitimizer of their age; similarly, the struggle for Mental Health and against Mental Illness is the grand legitimizer of ours.

6

Mental Illness and Mental Incompetence

The madman is not the man who has lost his reason. The madman is the man who has lost everything except his reason.
—Gibert K. Chesterton, *Orthodoxy*

Every organized system of human relations is, figuratively speaking, a game. To make such games work, the players must make certain tacit assumptions about each other. Thus, economists postulate an "economic man," who engages in rationally calculated relations of exchange with his fellows. One person may sell a bushel of wheat for ten dollars, another for a gun, a third for a handful of colored beads. Such exchange relations are reciprocal, each party playing the roles of both buyer and seller. Absent fraud, economists assume that each player acts rationally—that is, sells X in exchange for Y, because he prefers having Y to having X. For the most part, our economic relations continue to be based on such an assumption of rationality—which is why persons *under the age of contract* ("infants"), and those *beyond the pale of contract* ("idiots and the insane") are, a priori, excluded from playing that game.

I articulate this familiar assumption about economic relations to dramatize the contrast between it and the assumption underlying psychiatric relations—which are quintessentially nonreciprocal, resting on the assumption that one of the parties to the transaction is irrational and incompetent. Simply put, the psychiatrist is considered rational (until proven otherwise), while the patient is considered irrational (until proven otherwise). The terms *rational-irrational* in the previous sentence may, of course, be replaced with *sane-insane, competent-incompetent.*

Presumptions of this sort are most familiar to us in the rules governing the administration of the criminal law. To make a system of criminal justice work, it is necessary to presume that a person accused of an offense is innocent until proven guilty, or guilty until proven innocent.

111

We, Americans, are accustomed to our right to be presumed innocent—
and are justly proud of it, because it protects innocent persons accused
of crimes. In contrast, our rules governing psychiatric hospitalization and
treatment are based on the opposite premise—namely, that once a person
is called a "mental patient" he is presumed to be incompetent until proven
competent, and we are proud of this system, too, because it protects
incompetent persons from being burdened with the responsibility that
goes with competence. What is going on here? How can being denominated a "mental patient" transform a person, at one fell swoop, from being
considered a competent adult with rights into an incompetent patient
without any rights, save the "right" to be treated as a mental patient?

After more than three hundred years of psychiatric practice, people in
Western societies have become accustomed to assuming that sane persons are competent (until proven otherwise), and that insane persons,
called "mental patients," are incompetent (until proven otherwise). Although this denigrating presumption about the mental patient's moral
responsibility and legal accountability is anything but a secret, modern
mental health policies—based on the pretense that "mental illness is like
any other illness"—stubbornly fail to confront it. As a result, instead of
alleviating our confusion about the nature of mental illness and the moral
status of the mentally ill person, our social policies aggravate it. Perhaps
the single most important issue now facing the would-be mental-health
policymaker is, therefore, whether to presume that persons called "mentally ill" or "mental patients" are competent or incompetent?

In the bygone days of asylum psychiatry, such a question did not even
arise. If a person was mad enough to merit confinement in an insane
asylum, then he was manifestly incompetent; whereas if he was competent, then he was manifestly not a fit subject for incarceration in an insane
asylum and hence was not considered to be a mental patient at all. The
advent of outpatient psychiatric practice—that is, psychiatric (psychotherapeutic) practice in the physician's private office—radically altered
this situation. With the practice of psychoanalysis and other forms of
psychotherapies—conducted away from mental institutions—a new
class of mental patients entered the psychiatric scene: namely, the voluntary, ostensibly competent, patient. This development greatly enlarged
the range of psychiatric services available in Western societies; at the
same time, it hugely complicated and confused the legal relations between psychiatrists and mental patients. The upshot is that, today, psy-

chiatrists consider some mental patients competent, and others incompetent. How do they distinguish one from the other? The answer is that, for the most part, psychiatrists assign mental patients into one or another group depending on prevailing legal fashions and their own convenience, as the following revealing example illustrates.

On 7 December 1981, a man named Darrell Burch was found wandering along a Florida highway, appearing to be hurt and disoriented.

He was taken to Apalachee County Mental Health Services (ACMHS) in Tallahassee. . . . Its staff in their evaluation forms stated that, upon arrival at ACMHS, Burch was hallucinating, confused, and psychotic and believed he was "in heaven." . . . Burch was asked to sign forms giving his consent to admission and treatment. He did so. . . . [T]he facility's staff diagnosed his condition as paranoid schizophrenia and gave him psychotropic medication.[1]

Subsequently, Burch was transferred to the Florida State Hospital (FSH) in Chattahoochee, and was asked to sign, and signed, more forms giving consent to hospitalization and treatment at that institution. At the FSH, "Doctor Zinermon [a staff physician], wrote a 'progress note' indicating that Burch was 'refusing to cooperate' [and] would not answer questions . . ."[2] Burch remained at the FSH, as a "voluntary" patient, for five months. After he was released, Burch complained that he did not remember signing any forms, was mentally incompetent to consent to hospitalization and treatment, and sued Zinermon and ten other staff members of the FSH for having deprived him of liberty without due process of law. The defendants, he alleged,

knew or should have known that Plaintiff was incapable of voluntary, knowing, understanding, and informed consent to admission and treatment . . . Nonetheless, Defendants . . . seized plaintiff and against Plaintiff's will confined and imprisoned him and subjected him to involuntary treatment for the period from December 10, 1981, to May 7, 1982.[3]

The case went all the way to the Supreme Court, which ruled that when Burch was admitted to the FSH, he was incompetent and hence had a constitutionally protected right to a court hearing to determine whether he should be committed and treated as an involuntary patient. In other words, had Burch been formally committed, he would not have been deprived of liberty *without* due process, and hence his incarceration would have constituted hospitalization, not imprisonment. (Burch did not contest, but on the contrary affirmed, the validity of Florida's commitment laws.) Although this charade rests on the fiction of mental illness, it is not as illogical as it might seem. The Court explained its decision thus:

> The Florida statutes, of course, do not allow incompetent persons to be admitted as "voluntary" patients. . . . A patient who is willing to sign forms but incapable of informed consent certainly cannot be relied on to protest his "voluntary" admission and demand that the involuntary placement procedure be followed. The staff are the *only* persons in a position to take notice of any misuse of the voluntary admission procedure and to ensure that the proper procedure is followed.[4]

I do not know why the Justices of the Supreme Court decided to hear this case. But it seems to me that the reason might have been because they wished to reaffirm the classic, Kraepelinian principle that mental hospitalization ought to rest on the premise that anyone mentally sick enough to require it is—or ought to be presumed to be—mentally incompetent. Which is precisely what the Court said:

> [T]he very nature of mental illness makes it foreseeable that a person needing mental health care will be unable to understand any proffered "explanation and disclosure of the subject matter" of the forms that the person is asked to sign, and will be unable "to make a knowing and willing decision" whether to consent to admission. . . . The characteristics of mental illness thus create special problems regarding informed consent. Even if the State usually might be justified in taking at face value a person's request for admission to a hospital for *medical treatment*, it may not be justified in doing so, without further inquiry, as to a *mentally ill person's* request for admission and treatment at a *mental hospital*.[5]

In view of the fact that once a person is admitted to a mental hospital, he is stigmatized as crazy and cannot leave the premises at will, the Court's ruling is a welcome refutation of the mental health establishment's mendacious propaganda that "mental illness is like any other illness." In *Zinermon*, then, the Supreme Court acknowledges that, to paraphrase Samuel Goldwyn, anyone who seeks admission to a mental hospital ought to have his head examined. Unfortunately, the public remains unaware of the fact that the Supreme Court recognizes that voluntary mental hospitalization is a myth.

Not surprisingly, the Court's ruling upset the psychiatric establishment. Bruce J. Winick—a professor of law at the University of Miami—complained that "the Court's language could have unintended antitherapeutic consequences."[6] This cliché assumes that the purpose of incarcerating insane persons is therapy rather than tutelage—which is patently false. Specifically, Winick worried that,

If *Zinermon's* language is read this broadly, existing practices concerning voluntary admission will need substantial reexamination, and it is possible that the informal voluntary admission process could be transformed into a formal process resembling current practices for involuntary hospitalization.[7]

Although acknowledging that mental hospitalization is *inherently* involuntary is a far cry from abolishing psychiatric slavery, making that legal fact crystal clear to the public would be a step in that direction.

In this connection it is worth pointing out that what the medical and psychiatric community now views as a scientific advance from descriptive to biological psychiatry is only an escalation of deceit and hypocrisy concerning the legal status of the mental patient. I say this because—albeit, in *Zinermon*, the Supreme Court ignores the subject—until relatively recently (especially in Britain) the law provided three distinct options for admitting patients to mental hospitals: Admission could be voluntary, involuntary, or nonprotesting. The status of the involuntary patient was never in doubt. However, the majority of mental patients admitted as voluntary patients were, in fact—and still are—not voluntary in any meaningful sense of that term; instead, they were and are nonprotesting patients. As recently as 1968, an American Bar Foundation study acknowledged this important truth. Characterizing the nonprotesting patient as one who "acquiesces to hospitalization, neither taking the initiative himself nor resisting the initiative of others,"[8] the authors of the study emphasized that not many patients truly seek admission to mental hospitals, and few qualify as being "so dangerous or irresponsible that others must hospitalize [them]. . . . Most patients . . . do not object to hospitalization, but neither are they able to take the initiative in seeking it."[9] In thus recognizing the nonprotesting patient, the law at least tacitly acknowledged that the ambivalent and passive person also makes a kind of choice—he chooses to not protest.

Modern psychiatrists and medical ethicists dismiss the older psychiatry as "descriptive" and ostensibly reject the view that every mental (hospital) patient is, ipso facto, incompetent. It may thus come as a surprise that, in fact, contemporary psychiatrists and their allies continue to embrace the same presumption of incompetence. The following statement by Michael Moore, professor of law at the University of Pennsylvania and a recognized authority on mental health and the law, is typical:

Since mental illness negates our assumptions of rationality, we do not hold the mentally ill responsible. . . . [By] being unable to regard them as fully rational beings, we cannot affirm the essential condition to viewing them as moral agents to begin with.[10]

Clearly, in this context, the adjectives *irrational, incompetent, irresponsible*, and *mentally ill* are synonymous.

Ruth Macklin, a prominent medical ethicist, justifies coercive psychiatric paternalism with this assertion:

> I will argue . . . that if individual autonomy is a value that should be protected, promoted, and preserved, libertarians should recognize that autonomy may be lost by a patient's refusal of psychiatric treatment—treatment that might have prevented deterioration, humiliation, or decline.[11]

However, this sort of person usually rejects not only what Macklin calls psychiatric treatment, but the patient role itself. The argument thus rests on begging the question of how a free, criminally unindicted, American adult becomes a denominated, involuntary, mental patient. Notice, too, that Macklin says that "autonomy may be lost" as a result of refusing psychiatric treatment—a phrase that cloaks a linguistic blunder or subterfuge. When a physician offers a patient a treatment, the latter is faced with a choice between accepting or rejecting the procedure. The act of choosing is, *by definition*, an exercise of autonomy. To be sure, the result of such a choice may be not only loss of autonomy, but loss of life itself. But unless we assume that the chooser's autonomy is already impaired (by mental illness) and hence is not the exercise of "true" autonomy, the argument has no force. To make matters worse, Macklin also claims that in her argument "nothing whatever hangs on whether mental illness is a myth,"[12] an assertion utterly inconsistent with her repeated use of psychiatric scenarios and her acceptance of the legitimacy of specifically *psychiatric* coercion. For example, she refers to persons with "manic flights" who are difficult to deal with because "they enjoy the hypermanic experience. . . . Such people could be said to be wholly lacking in autonomy when in those states."[13] Macklin's reasoning is thus self-contradictory: The person denominated as (severely) mentally ill is presumed to lack autonomy (competence), yet has a choice of refusing treatment and thereby losing his autonomy; hence, it is justified to treat him against his (expressed) wishes, because doing so will preserve and restore his autonomy. This reasoning assumes not only that the behaviors called "mental illnesses" are diseases, an assumption Macklin denies, but also that the risk-benefit ratio of every intervention called "psychiatric treatment" is such that a rational person would *always* choose treatment rather than nontreatment. In short, however the argument in support of involuntary psychiatric interventions may be framed, it presents us with the classic, legal-psychiatric premise that it is medically and morally right to treat persons denominated as mental patients against their will—because they are like children. Examples abound.

A sixty-year-old Salt Lake City woman takes Halcion, shoots her mother to death, has the criminal charges against her dropped on the ground that she was mentally incompetent at the time of the shooting, sues Upjohn Company which manufactures Halcion, and collects an undisclosed amount in an out-of-court settlement.[14] How could this happen? It could happen because the claimant did not have to prove that she was incompetent at the time she shot her mother, or that her incompetence was caused by Halcion; it was enough that she was defined as a mental patient, and that two psychiatrists testified that she was "involuntarily intoxicated when she shot her 83-year-old mother."[15] In other words, the jury's presumption was that when this woman shot her mother, she was (acutely) mentally ill and incompetent. The burden of proof thus fell upon the defendant, the Upjohn Company (with deep pockets in its capitalist robes), to show that the woman was not mentally ill, was not mentally incompetent, and that Halcion did not cause her to shoot her mother.

Despite the popularity of this paternalistic-psychiatric prejudice, the suspicion lingers that there may be method in madness—that one man's rationality may be another's irrationality. An interesting example of such skepticism, which nevertheless refrains from confronting psychiatry's favorite fictions, is *Choice and Consequence*, by Thomas C. Schelling, a professor of political economy at Harvard. The index to this 350-page book lists topics such as drug addiction, health-related issues, and gambling, but has no entry for illness, insanity, mental illness, or psychiatry. Regarding the question of who is rational, Schelling writes: "The critical question is not whether a person is 'rational' according to any particular definition, perfectionist or merely approximate, but whether his choice is determined in large part by the situation he is in and by what we can guess about his values."[16] This seems to me a pretentious rephrasing of Shakespeare's oft-quoted assertion that there is method in madness.

How can even serious thinkers differ so profoundly about whether or not mentally ill persons are competent and responsible for their actions? I believe the answer lies in the fact that we treat words such as *rational* and *competent* as if they described a person's capacity or condition (which they may), when in fact we deploy them as injunctions to justify adopting a particular stance toward him.[17] Consider, for example, the question: Is an intelligent seventeen-year-old competent to make binding contracts? If we use the term *competent* to describe a person's ability to do something—as when we speak of a person as a competent skier or tennis player—then a seventeen-year-old may, of course, be competent. In fact, he is likely to be a more competent basketball player or runner than his father or mother. However, if we use the term injunctively—to identify the sort of legal attitude we, as adults, must maintain in our economic or sexual relationships with him—then a seventeen-year-old is, by definition, not competent. In short, the crux of the confusion lies in that psychiatrists typically use the term *competent* as if they were identifying a mental quality *in* the designated person, when in fact they are advocating a particular attitude *toward him*.

These considerations explain the contradiction between Shakespeare's view of insane persons as competent, and Freud's view of them as incompetent. Although, at bottom, there is little difference between what these men had to say about human nature, there is a vast difference between the attitude each took up vis-a-vis the mad person. Shakespeare viewed Lady Macbeth as "Not so sick . . . as troubled with thick-coming fancies," for which she "More needs . . . the divine than the physician,"[18] whereas Freud viewed her as suffering from a bona fide disease susceptible to bona fide treatments. The same division lies at the heart of the controversy between Freud and Jung. Freud wanted to turn the study and treatment of madness into a positivistic, scientific affair, while Jung wanted to return it to the domain of morals and religion.[19]

Indeed, if one reads between the lines of psychiatric treatises, one discovers that psychiatrists sometimes frankly admit that their ostensibly medical determinations and diagnoses are, in fact, disguises for certain tactical decisions and recommendations. For example, Ivor Batchelor, the author of the prestigious *Henderson and Gillespie's Textbook of Psychiatry*, writes:

> We suggest that in dealing with such matters [the criminal responsibility of offenders] the same *tactics* should be employed as in all other branches of medical and social

work—to prevent criminal conduct, and any accompanying mental disorder from developing, rather than to attempt the somewhat futile task of remedying it after it has become fully established.[20]

For the most part, then, psychiatric deliberations about competence conceal dispositional decisions behind seemingly scientific determinations.

Although it is clear that the policy of declaring a person incompetent to stand trial rests on the use of a pseudomedical concept as a rhetorical justification for a legal disposition, the fact remains that certain bodily injuries and illnesses can, and do, impair or annul a person's competence. I want to briefly consider these conditions and their legal consequences.

The Anglo-American legal system affords elaborate procedural protections to persons accused of crime—one of them being the right to defend oneself in court. Suppose, then, that in the course of an armed robbery, the burglar is shot in the head by a policeman. The accused lies in bed in a hospital, unconscious. Plainly, it would be unfair to try him in that condition. Accordingly, the trial is postponed until the defendant is "fit to stand trial."[21]

The policy of protecting mentally ill persons from standing trial rests on the same premise. "As a matter of fairness and humanity," wrote the great English jurist, William Blackstone in 1765, the trial of an "insane defendant" must be postponed until he is able to "make his own defense."[22] This immediately plunges us back into the problem of insanity, into what "it" is and how we determine whether a person has or has not got "it." I have said enough about this subject and will say no more about it here. Instead, I shall only show that, by basing a policy on the fundamentally faulty idea that a metaphoric illness is a real (literal) disease, we have created a policy that serves a purpose diametrically opposed to the purpose it was ostensibly intended to serve.

Illness—say, cancer of the colon—is a fact. Mental illness "causing" incompetence to stand trial—say, the alleged incompetence of Ezra Pound—is a claim. The bullet wound and unconsciousness of the hypothetical burglar shot in the head are facts; nevertheless, his inability to stand trial is a claim, albeit one that rests on his physical impairment. This distinction is crucial, because while a fact may "speak for itself," a claim must be advanced by an individual, on his own behalf or on behalf of another person. In the case of the unconscious burglar, the claim of his inability to stand trial would be advanced by an attorney, and would be supported by physicians. Sometimes—for example, in the case of a person suffering from heart disease—the defendant might himself claim that he is unable (not mentally incompetent) to stand trial. My point is that, in our present medico-legal system, it is inconceivable that a conscious person, not considered to be mentally ill, would be declared incompetent to stand trial against his will—on the basis of bodily illness and the testimony of (nonpsychiatric) physicians to that effect. Who could or would advance such a claim? The defendant's attorney could not do so, because the defendant would simply fire him if he did. The defendant's physician could not do so, because there would be no one to solicit his opinion, which could therefore not come to the court's attention. The court could not do so, because judges have not (yet) taken it upon themselves to "protect" bodily ill persons from the hazards of appearing in court. In the case of mental illness, the whole situation is not merely different, but all the assumptions and rules are inverted: As I indicated, (severe) mental illness is regarded not only as a bona fide disease (like heart disease), but also as a *prima facie* case of mental incompetence (like unconsciousness).

There are certain other situations in which a person may, de facto, be unable to assist in his own defense and hence be unfit to stand trial. The most common conditions that may cause mental incompetence are injuries (especially to the head) and intoxications severe enough to render the subject unconscious. By definition, an unconscious person is unable to assist in his own defense, hence incompetent—to stand trial or consent to medical care. His incapacity to make such a determination is apparent even to untrained observers. Still another class of incapacitating conditions are the deliria—manifestations of disturbances of brain function without loss of consciousness, typically caused by injury, intoxication, or infection. Although deliria are behavioral manifestations of brain disease, the presence of underlying brain disease can be inferred from objective findings demonstrated by means of blood or spinal fluid tests, electroencephalography, and skull X rays. A delirious person is unable to care for himself and is thus properly treated as incompetent.

Because the delirious person and the so-called mental patient both exhibit what the normal observer calls "irrational behavior," psychiatrists and lay persons alike are inclined to view the latter also as if he suffered from the former condition (whose nature, qua delirium, is not yet objectively demonstrable). This, of course, is a variation on the theme of interpreting mental illness as bodily illness. To appreciate the weakness of the analogy, we must consider the similarities and the differences between the delirious person and the psychotic person.

Actually, the only similarity between the delirious-incompetent and the mentally ill-incompetent person is that both behave inappropriately and upset others. In every other way, they and their conditions differ. Unlike the delirious person, the mentally ill person suffers from no demonstrable disease; indeed, he is typically eager to chart his own course in life, however ill-advised that course may be to him or others. In addition, more often than not, he can find friends, doctors, and lawyers to support his choices, represent him in court, and testify on his behalf. I have chronicled the fate of several persons, some quite famous, who have been declared mentally incompetent to stand trial despite their own protestations against such a categorization, and despite the fact that lawyers and psychiatrists supported their claims of being competent.[23]

Nevertheless, if the media convince the public that the subject is mentally ill—as the American media did in the case of Ezra Pound, for example—then the procedure is validated as legitimate, the psychiatric protection of a mentally incompetent individual. However, if psychiatrists use the same tactic in a Communist country, and if the media categorizes the victim as a "dissident," then we regard the procedure as illegitimate, the paradigm of a "psychiatric abuse." This is foolish. In both cases, the outcome is the inexorable consequence of the concept of mental incompetence *due* to mental illness: If a person is psychiatrically diagnosed as "mentally incompetent," and judicially declared to be "incompetent to stand trial," then, ipso facto, he must also be incompetent to decide whether he wants to advance that claim in court or retain counsel or psychiatrists to represent him. These decisions must therefore be made *for* the mentally ill person by others, often with devastating consequences. Why must the consequences of such a policy be harmful for the so-called incompetent patient? Because he is denied the right to trial, guaranteed by the Sixth Amendment to the Constitution, and is incarcerated in a psychiatric institution. Indeed, prior to 1972—when the Supreme Court recognized the grave abuses that this policy had spawned and placed strict limits on its application—even defendants charged with minor offenses often ended up spending the rest of their lives imprisoned, without trial, in hospitals for the criminally insane.[24]

Ironically, because the American system of criminal justice is so intensely concerned with protecting innocent persons from punishment, it has proved especially vulnerable to corruption by excuses couched in terms of psychiatric disabilities. The reasons for this tragedy may be briefly summarized as follows.

One of the root concepts of Anglo-American law is *mens rea*, a doctrine that holds that unlawful behavior constitutes a crime only if it is committed by an actor who possesses a "guilty mind." At least since the late Middle Ages, insane persons have been regarded as lacking *mens rea*. In fact, one would be justified in turning this relationship around and asserting, with William Blackstone, that the root of the modern concept of insanity is the absence of *mens rea*: "All the several pleas and excuses which protect the committer of a forbidden act from punishment which is otherwise annexed thereto may be reduced to a single consideration: the want or defect of *will*."[25] This is why children and mental patients— "infants, idiots, and the insane," in John Locke's language—are not prosecuted or punished by the criminal law, but instead are restrained, as minors and as mad, by family courts and mental health laws. However, the analogy between children and the insane fails to take account of the fact that childhood is an objectively defined chronological condition, but insanity is not. Moreover, since children are under tutelage, whereas (normal) adults are not, the analogy between children and the insane begs the question of which adults should be placed under tutelage, for what reasons, and for how long.

Scrutiny of the implications of insanity as an excusing condition for crime reveals additional difficulties. To begin with, the concept of *mens rea* qua mental competence implies a distinction between competence to commit a crime and competence to commit an unlawful act. Thus, a person who possesses *mens rea* is viewed as competent to commit an unlawful act that is a crime, whereas one who lacks *mens rea* is viewed as competent to commit only an unlawful act, but not a crime. But this easily leads to a contradiction. Inasmuch as our view of competence to commit an unlawful act is similar to our view of practical competence (say, to play the piano), it follows that a person considered incompetent to commit an unlawful act ought also to be considered incompetent to enter a plea or to stand trial for the unlawful act-qua-crime. Of course, there is no such consistency in the use of the idea of insanity in the criminal justice system. The result is caprice, confusion, and injustice on a truly colossal scale.

For example, a defendant pleading insanity is considered to be competent to plead: He is permitted to plead—guilty, not guilty, or not guilty by reason of insanity; and he is allowed to stand trial. Nevertheless, if his insanity defense is "successful," he is retroactively regarded as having been insane at the time of the unlawful act, and hence incompetent to have committed a crime. This conclusion generates a host of increasingly more absurd questions, such as: When the trial begins, is the defendant still insane, or has he recovered his sanity between the commission of the unlawful act and the time of the trial? (If he has not, he should not have been allowed to plead and stand trial.) When the trial ends, is the defendant insane, even though he was considered competent to plead and stand trial?

If the jury rejects the plea of insanity and finds the defendant guilty, other ambiguities of the meaning of insanity-qua-incompetence surface. If having a mental illness—like having diabetes or pneumonia—is a factual (medical) matter, as psychiatrists maintain, then how can a jury determine its presence or absence? The usual answer begs the question by taking advantage of the ambiguity inherent in the dual, factual-and-dispositional, dimensions of the insanity plea. In short, both legal and medical experts can fall back on the claim that a lay jury neither affirms nor denies medical findings, which it lacks the competence to do; instead, it decides whether the insanity-defendant "deserves" to be punished or treated, a judgment considered to lie within the ken of a lay jury. But this will not do, because the "successful" insanity acquittee ends up in a mental hospital for the treatment of his mental illness—a (supposedly) judicial disposition thus resulting in (officially) medical consequences.

Two other basic concepts related to mental competence that enter into our thinking about, and formulations of, mental health policy need to be briefly mentioned: namely, consent and contract. The concept of consent—to examination, testing, treatment, and so forth—is clearly contingent on competence. In a medical context, the most important consequential meaning of competence is that a person deemed competent has the right to assume or reject the patient role; and that, even after he has assumed the patient role, he retains the right to consent to, or withhold consent from, being subjected to particular diagnostic and therapeutic interventions. For example, as a rule, a Jehovah's Witness is considered to be competent—and can therefore request, and may be granted the option of—receiving surgical treatment without a blood transfusion.

Whereas consent is unilateral, something an actor grants another or withholds from him—contract is reciprocal, a compact between two or more parties for performing mutually agreed-upon acts (services). The concepts of competence and consent refer to one person only—in the medical context, to the patient. Contract introduces the physician into the relationship: Patient and physician harmonize their wishes and cooperate on agreed-upon terms.

In everyday language, the word *contract* means an agreement between two or more persons to do, or to refrain from doing, something—typically, delivering certain goods or services in exchange for money. A contract is a bargain, a compact, a covenant, a promise. In legal theory, contract is defined as a set of promises protected from breach by law, a definition that recognizes that a contract may be broken, and, if it is broken, the party who breaks it owes certain remedies to the party he has injured.

The idea of a binding, mutually enforceable contract is perhaps the single most important element of modern, market-oriented (capitalist) societies. Of course, there are many non-contractual arrangements for producing and distributing goods and services—such as, slavery, serfdom, paternalism, socialism, and communism. Let us try to be clear about the advantages and disadvantages of contractual and noncontractual arrangements for providing health-care services.

The principal value of contractual health-care arrangements is that they maximize and protect the freedom of action of both the patient and the doctor. In a contractual medical (psychiatric) context, a person becomes a patient only if and when he wants to, just as he becomes a customer for buying automobiles or houses only if and when he wants to; and a physician becomes the dispenser of medical care for a particular patient only if and when he wants to. Accordingly, only in such a context are both patient and physician free to reject each other as well as to refuse to become parties to certain (unwanted) medical interventions—such as abortion or electroshock. Contract also protects each party from the contract violations of his partner: The patient is free to fire his doctor, and the doctor is free to reject treating a person he does not want as his patient. We must keep these seemingly obvious features of contractual health-care arrangements in mind, because when people seek to protect choice (as individual liberty and personal responsibility), they regard reciprocal contractual limitations as the system's supreme strength—but when they seek to protect people from the dangers of mental illness, they regard such limitations as its fatal flaw. To understand this fundamental self-contradiction, we must briefly reconsider the concepts of competence and consent.

Although the classic psychoanalytic relationship, and other psychotherapeutic relationships based on it, rest on contract, they are the exceptions to the psychiatric rule. Institutional psychiatry has always been, and continues to be, based not on consent and contract, but on paternalism and coercion. The ideal role of the psychiatric physician is similar to that of a protective parent, and the role of the psychiatric (hospital) patient is similar to that of a misbehaving child—the latter being properly subjected to the authority and care of his guardian. Looking over both protector and protected, supervising their relationship to each other and to the community, stands the Therapeutic State: It authorizes the psychiatrist's coercion of the patient, and it supplies the force and funds needed to ensure the patient's compliance with the psychiatric rules. The patient is thus freed of the burden of contracting with the psychiatrist and gains subtle powers to coerce him—by means of "symptoms." *Mutatis mutandis*, the psychiatrist is freed of the burden of contracting with his patient and gains not-so-subtle powers to coerce him—by means of commitment, compulsory treatment, and the threats of such interventions. What both lose in the bargain is, of course, freedom and responsibility.[26]

I have tried to show that competence, consent, and contract are interrelated concepts, forming a progressive series, as it were. Remove competence, and the conditions for both consent and contract are negated; remove consent, and the conditions for contract are negated; remove contract, and the conditions for freedom and responsibility are negated.

Ostensibly, recent (so-called) reforms in mental-health policy have been generated by the desire to free the mental patient from old-fashioned, authoritarian psychiatric controls. As a result, certain forms of crass psychiatric coercions, such as easy and indefinite involuntary mental hospitalization, have become unfashionable. But recent changes in mental health policy have utterly failed to increase the mental patients' responsibility to care for himself, to be accountable for his everyday behavior, and to be legally answerable for his criminal conduct. On the contrary, more people than ever are now defined as mental patients and continue to be cared for and treated paternalistically, without their consent, as if they were incompetent. It is indeed possible that some people cannot be treated contractually, because they refuse to commit themselves to binding promises. Whether or on what terms a particular mental patient is willing to make contracts is an empirical question; moreover, it is much easier to answer that question than the question of what kind of illness afflicts him and how he might be cured of it. For my part, I remain persuaded that we cannot make progress in mental health care policy (in the sense of reducing the proportion of persons in the population treated as insane and incompetent), until we relinquish our obsession with mental illness as a supposedly medical condition "in" the patient, and instead confront the strategic uses to which we, nonpatients, put this idea, and acknowledge the practical benefits its use provides for us.[27]

7

The Illusion of Mental Patients' Rights

*The greatest detriment to the mentally ill may be
the "patients rights" laws.*
—Families of the Mentally Ill Collective,
Families Helping Families Living with Schizophrenia

During the past quarter of a century, "the rights of mental patients"
has been a popular topic in both the specialized literature of mental health
and law, and in the popular press. Indeed, the subject has attracted the
attention of even the United Nations, as an area in which human rights
and ostensibly therapeutic practices are on a collision course.[1]

Where does the idea of giving rights to, or guaranteeing the rights of,
mental patients come from? It comes from two sources: the long legal-
psychiatric tradition of depriving mental patients of rights; and the recent
fashion—ostensibly civil libertarian, but actually bureaucratic-statist—
of giving rights to members of special groups of "victims," such as
blacks, women, and homosexuals.

Before going further, I want to emphasize that liberty is a matter of
law and political philosophy—not therapy; that illness is a matter of
pathology—not psychopathology; that the connection between rights
and diseases is a matter of social convention—not science; and that, in
the American political tradition, human beings are considered to possess
civil rights because they are persons—not because they are members of
special groups.

Prior to this century, the term *civil rights* meant limits on state power
as a means of protecting the individual from coercion by the state.
Somewhere down the line, the phrase underwent an Orwellian metamorphosis and came to mean the moral legitimacy of a special interest group,
such as blacks or women, using the power of the state to impose its
demands on the rest of the people. Although this metamorphosis has had

127

some undesirable effects on blacks and women, those most adversely affected by it have, not surprisingly, been mental patients.

I say not surprisingly because, according to conventional wisdom, the insane are irrational and hence do not recognize their own needs and rights. Who, then, should speak for them? More than thirty years ago, when I began to address the problem of the rights of persons called "mentally ill," I emphasized that I speak for myself only. I also noted that since many different kinds of persons are called mental patients, they cannot all have the same interests; and that, in any case, they can and should speak for themselves. As for what is now called "mental health advocacy," I have stood firmly for the policy of viewing mental patients as persons, presumed competent and innocent until proven otherwise, who ought to be treated by the law with the same disregard for their psychiatric status as for their religious status.

Since then, essentially the opposite has actually happened. Rallying to the battle cry of "civil rights for mental patients," professional civil libertarians and the relatives of mental patients joined conventional psychiatrists demanding rights for mental patients, qua mental patients. The result has been a perverse sort of affirmative action program: Because mental patients are ill, they have a right to treatment; because many are homeless, they have a right to housing; and so it goes, until mental patients have a profusion of nominal rights, but no real rights at all. Do I exaggerate? Consider the evidence. The state of New York has a bureaucracy called the New York State Commission on Quality of Care for the Mentally Disabled. The commission has a program, called Protection and Advocacy for Mentally Ill Individuals (PAMII), which in turn publishes a pamphlet that explains its mandate as "help[ing] people whose rights are being threatened." The pamphlet then asks: "WHAT RIGHTS?", and offers the following list in reply:

The right not to be physically, sexually, or verbally abused
The right not to receive "inappropriate or excessive medical treatment"
The right to participate in and approve your treatment plan
The right to accept or refuse treatment and to be informed about the treatment you are offered
The right to the most appropriate treatment in the least restrictive setting
The right to privacy and confidentiality
The right to review your medical records
The right to make a complaint without fear of retaliation
The right to financial entitlements
    and many more . . .[2]

Of course, these are rights that every non-mental patient has without special dispensation from his protectors. In short, the phrase, *the rights of mental patients*, has come to mean anything and everything but one thing—namely, according mental patients the same rights as are accorded all adults qua persons.

A recent British study, titled "The Rights of Mentally Ill People," exemplifies both the futility of trying to secure rights for mental patients qua mental patients, and the uncomprehending stubbornness with which this quest is now pursued throughout the English-speaking world. Prepared by Chris Heginbotham—the national director of the National Association for Mental Health of England and Wales, and a board member of the World Federation for Mental Health—the report also illustrates that the professional protectors of the rights of mental patients are just as great a threat to their rights as the psychiatrists against whom these self-appointed guardians propose to guard them. Heginbotham begins by asserting that "people with mental illnesses are a disadvantaged ... minority in every country." Then, in characteristic collectivistic-statist style, he confuses needs and rights and equates the one with the other: "This Report concentrates primarily on the *needs* of people defined as having a diagnosable mental disorder."[3]

But ignoring an adult's wants and pontificating about his needs renders attending to his rights virtually impossible. Thus, when Heginbotham uses the word *right*, he means not the traditional, legal right to be left alone but, the modern, political right to make demands on others. Asserting that "it can reasonably be argued that every person has the right to be treated according to the following principles," Heginbotham proceeds to enumerate the goods and services persons who qualify as victims ought to be given:

> To a large extent this report is concerned with rights—the right of people with diagnosable mental illnesses to be treated with "equal concern and respect." ... This must include the right to receive proper care, support, and treatment for any illness, physical or mental.[4]

After contemptuously dismissing the view "that the term 'mental illness' is ... a myth,"[5] Heginbotham proceeds, without further discussion, to adopt the World Health Organization's definition of mental illness and its estimate of its incidence: "A rough estimate suggests that at any time no less than 40 million people—perhaps as many as 100 million—in the world are suffering from the most serious mental disorders as defined by WHO."[6]

That takes care of the problem of what mental illness *is*, and of how many people have got it. With these matters out of the way, Heginbotham comes down squarely in support of conventional psychiatric interventions. He writes: "The release of these people [involuntarily hospitalized patients], admirable in theory, has often been disastrous in practice. A recent sample survey of New York's homeless found that 96% had at one time been in a psychiatric hospital."[7]

This is a careless and prejudiced way to talk about deinstitutionalization. Does Heginbotham argue that deinstitutionalization has been disastrous for the patients—even if they prefer to be out of the hospital at any cost? Or that it has been disastrous for the patients' families—especially if they prefer to keep the patients in the hospital at any cost? Or that it has been disastrous for the people in the cities whom they annoy and disturb—and who have nothing to gain by deinstitutionalization? Heginbotham does not say. He also does not ask who considers deinstitutionalization to be a failure. The patients who prefer to be out of mental hospitals? The patients who prefer to be in mental hospitals? The patients' relatives? Obviously, the answers vary, if for no other reason than because these parties often have conflicting interests, which Heginbotham systematically fails to acknowledge.

One of the many ironies of the "mental patients' rights movement" is the way its rhetoric fits so perfectly the collectivistic-paternalistic spirit of traditional Oriental despotism and twentieth-century communism. Indeed, the Soviets—always a soft touch for the statist mentality that eagerly relinquishes real personal freedoms in return for fictitious legal rights—have joined the parade of giving persons defamed as mental patients rights, the better to justify taking away their liberties. In January 1988, Tass reported the enactment of a set of psychiatric reforms, among them a law making it a crime "to lock up a patently healthy person in a mental hospital."[8] No psychiatrist who engaged in this practice prior to the enactment of this law was named. After all, no particular bureaucrat—political or psychiatric—is ever guilty of anything; only "the system" is guilty. In any case, the important thing is not to worry about past psychiatric abuses but to proclaim future guarantees against them, enshrined in new rights. American politicians, lawyers, and even civil libertarians are proud that American mental patients have rights; henceforth, Soviet mental patients will have exactly the same rights. The Tass report continued: "People receiving psychiatric assistance . . . are guaranteed legal aid by a lawyer with a view to ensuring their rights."[9]

No doubt, mental patients in the Soviet Union need all the rights they can get, and then some. Emboldened by *glasnost*, Sergei Grigoryants, chief editor of the magazine *Glasnost*, wrote: "According to official data, nearly five million people are listed on the psychiatric register in the Soviet Union. . . . To be on it officially permits a healthy person to be placed in a psychiatric *prison* at any time *and to be deprived of all rights*."[10] Of course, like all conventional critics of psychiatry, Grigoryants protests only against "healthy people" being forced to become the patients of psychiatrists he himself characterizes as "criminal[s] . . . defending [their] right to murder."[11] As I remarked elsewhere, it is mysterious what there is about mental illness that renders a person suffering from it a fit subject for compulsory care by murderers.[12]

I regard all this sound and fury as a collective exercise in deception and self-deception. Indeed, Grigoryants soon bit the Communist dust: On 19 May 1988, the *New York Times* reported that after having spent a week in jail, Grigoryants had been released and was charged with "defaming the Soviet state. . . . The authorities had confiscated his printing equipment and destroyed his files and manuscripts."[13] It is hard to see how one Soviet state agency could protect the rights of a person whose rights have been abrogated, presumably rightfully, by another state agency. Moreover, when the mental patient's right to liberty conflicts with his right to treatment—whether in the United States or in the USSR—what official, on the basis of what criteria, decides which right should prevail?

We cannot escape from this psychiatric trap of our own making. The ostensible aim of every involuntary psychiatric intervention is to treat a person for his mental illness; its actual result is that he is deprived of liberty. Similarly, the ostensible aim of every psychiatric reform is to make the mental health system less susceptible to abuse; its actual result is that the system and its abuses become more impregnable to criticism. Ironically, the promoters of psychiatric slavery—both in the United States and in the USSR—now employ the identical rhetoric of "dangerousness to self and others" to identify certain individuals as mental patients, and the identical justification of "patients' rights" to legitimize incarcerating them.

An important corollary of the notion that civil rights adhere to individuals qua persons, as against individuals qua members of one or another special group, is the conjoining of rights and responsibilities, liberties and duties. This is why, for hundreds of years, Anglo-American political philosophers exempted three groups of human beings from the class of full-fledged persons: infants, idiots, and the insane. Because children, retarded persons, and psychotics are considered to be unable to fulfill the social duties of normal adults (which some of them are indeed incapable of fulfilling), individuals assigned to these categories are deprived of rights and exempted from responsibilities.

Mutatis mutandis, because the rights and responsibilities of an individual cannot be disjoined (or can be disjoined only temporarily and to a very limited extent), the very idea of the rights of mental patients is a patent absurdity: How could a person be allowed to enjoy the privileges of individual liberty without any corresponding responsibility to obey the law? Because rights and responsibilities cannot—and, in fact, are not—so disjoined, I maintain that the words *mental patient* and *right* contradict each other and are mutually exclusive, just as Rousseau maintained that "the words *slave* and *right* contradict each other and are mutually exclusive."[14] It is ironic that while no one in Rousseau's day would have disagreed with his assertion about the oxymoronic character of attributing rights to slaves, hardly anyone today agrees with my assertion about the oxymoronic character of attributing rights to involuntarily hospitalized mental patients. Why is this so? How can people not see that the mental patient's right to treatment is, in fact, a hypocritical disguise for the psychiatrist's right to assault the patient—physically, chemically, electrically, and in every other way—and call it "treatment."[15] After pondering this question for a long time, I concluded that the answer probably lies in the secularization of the Roman Catholic Principle of Double Effect. Without ever mentioning this moral rule, perhaps without even being fully aware of it, many people—in and outside of the mental health professions—now support psychiatric slavery by falling back on a therapeutic (in)version of this classic, Thomistic idea.

Because Thomas Aquinas clearly articulated and firmly supported this particular form of moral reasoning, he is credited with its authorship. In his *Summa Theologica*, in the chapter titled "Whether It Is Lawful to Kill a Man in Self-Defense?" Aquinas justified the otherwise illicit act of killing a man as follows:

> Nothing hinders one act from having two effects, only one of which is intended, while the other is beside the intention. Now moral acts take their species according to what is intended, and not according to what is beside the intention. Accordingly, the act of self-defense may have two effects, one is the saving of one's life, the other is the slaying of the aggressor. Therefore this act, since one's intention is to save one's own life, is not unlawful.[16]

The *New Catholic Encyclopedia* defines the Principle of Double Effect as follows: "A rule of conduct frequently used in moral theology to determine when a person may lawfully perform an action from which two effects follow, one bad, the other good."[17] For example, it is considered permissible for a physician to give an aged patient a painkiller, provided the aim is to relieve pain, even though the effect may also be to hasten death. In contemporary Catholic analyses, this principle is often applied to such topics as abortion, contraception, and suicide.

Obviously, this mode of reasoning is in no sense peculiarly Catholic or restricted to Catholics. Anyone intent on rationalizing his own morally contradictory interests can make use of it, and many people do. For example, Paul Ramsey—said to be "the most influential American Protestant writer on medical ethics of his generation"—has applied it to the problem of abortion. David Smith, a professor of religious studies at the University of Indiana, approvingly cites Ramsey's work to support the proposition that "the love commandment is the basic rule or principle of Christian ethics. 'Everything [he quotes Ramsey] is lawful, *absolutely everything* is permitted which love permits, everything without a single exception. And *absolutely everything* is commanded which love requires, absolutely everything without the slightest exception or 'softening.'"[18] Utterances such as this make it clear why it has been so easy to enlist compassion and love on the side of the psychiatric battalions.[19] Smith then explains Ramsey's position on abortion as follows:

> [D]irect abortions are justified in situations where a nonviable fetus threatens its mother's life. In that case: the intention of the action, and in this sense its direction, is not upon the death of the fetus . . . [but is] directed toward the *incapacitation* of the fetus from doing what it is doing to the life of the mother. . . . This distinction between incapacitation and direct killing solves the problem of explaining how love can justify abortion. If justifiable abortions are properly described as incapacitating rather than killing, then one can say that such actions are justifiable actions of love to the aborted fetus. One has not done something unloving to the fetus itself.[20]

Truly, the human mind is not an organ of reasoning, but an organ of self-justification.

Reflecting about the forms into which the arguments for and against psychiatric deprivations of liberty have hardened, I have become persuaded that the Principle of Double Effect offers the correct angle from which to view the standoff. I present herewith, in schematic form, two hypothetical dialogues that may help us to transcend this impasse.

Concerning contraception:

CRITIC: You say you are a good Catholic and yet you take birth control pills. Your behavior proves that you are not a good Catholic. You are a hypocrite.

CATHOLIC WOMAN: You are wrong and unfair to me. There is nothing I want more than to have a baby. Besides, I don't take birth control pills; you describe what I do that way only to embarrass and humiliate me. I take a medicine prescribed for me by a physician to regulate my irregular and painful menstrual periods.

CRITIC: Regardless of what you say, the effect of the medicine you take is that you are less likely to become pregnant.

CATHOLIC WOMAN: That may be. But, I swear to God, that is not my intention. And I may get pregnant. As you know perfectly well, it is not at all certain that the medicine I take will prevent it.

Concerning commitment:

CRITIC: You say you are a humanist and love liberty and yet you incarcerate innocent persons. Your behavior proves that you are neither a humanist nor do you love liberty. You are a hypocrite.

PSYCHIATRIST: You are wrong and unfair to me. There is nothing I want more than to liberate my patients from the shackles of their mental illness. Besides, I don't incarcerate anyone; you describe what I do that way only to embarrass and humiliate me. I hospitalize patients to enable them to recover from their illnesses.

CRITIC: Regardless of what you say, the effect of your intervention is that your patient is deprived of liberty.

PSYCHIATRIST: That may be. But, I swear by Hippocrates, that is not my intention. Anyway, the patient will soon be discharged. And, as you know perfectly well, it is not at all certain that, after being discharged from the hospital, the patient will object to such a temporary loss of liberty.

Although these dialogues are imaginary, the situations they describe are not. It is important to add that although the Catholic Principle of Double Effect and the Psychiatric Principle of Double Effect appear to be similar, they are not the same; in fact, the latter is an inverted version of the former. In Catholic theology, the initial act cannot be morally evil, albeit some of its consequences might be: for example, self-defense is a right, even though it may cause the assailant's death, which is a wrong. In the psychiatric ethic, the initial act may be evil, so long as its consequence is not: for example, it is wrong to deprive a person of liberty, but it becomes right to do so if it cures him of mental illness. In short, in the Catholic ethic the means cannot be evil, although some of its consequences might be; whereas in the psychiatric ethic, good ends justify evil means.

This type of reasoning is now used to justify the incarceration and involuntary treatment of so-called street persons. Psychiatrists insists that homeless mentally ill persons are hospitalized against their will solely because they are ill, and not because they are homeless. For example, apropos of the forcible hospitalization of Joyce Brown, the New York bag lady who attracted much attention in the fall of 1987, Luis Marcos, a psychiatrist and vice president for mental health of the city's Health and Hospitals Corporation, declared:

> We are dealing with people who are severely mentally and physically ill. And people have a right to be treated and cared for. . . . The civil liberties unions believe people should be free to live in the street and to deteriorate. We believe people should be free from hallucinations and mental illness. She [Joyce Brown] was not hospitalized because she was living on the streets—she was hospitalized because in the judgment of at least three psychiatrists she needed medical psychiatric help.[21]

Does Marcos really believe that had Joyce Brown been living in a luxurious condominium on Park Avenue, on a tax-free annual income of $1 million, she would nevertheless have come to the attention of his roving psychiatrists cruising the streets looking for patients, much less that she would have been forcibly hospitalized in a public mental institution? In addition, Marcos's views are troubling because his remark that Joyce Brown "was not hospitalized because she was living on the streets" implies that she has a right to live on the streets. But does she? The question reminds one of Anatole France's famous protest that "the law, in its majestic equality, forbids the rich as well as the poor to sleep under bridges, to beg in the streets, and to steal bread."[22] This phrase, made immortal by generation after generation of socialists and statists, mocks precisely that equality before the law that Edmund Burke and every adherent to the rule of law before and since then has venerated. And with France's remark too, the question of credibility arises. Did he really believe that the poor should be allowed to steal bread? Surely, he must have known that such a rule would annul any rational person's decision to operate a bakery. The same principle applies to sleeping under bridges or on hot air grates: Allowing the poor to sleep on the sidewalks of New York would inevitably lead to no one—poor or rich—having the cultural and social amenities and protections everyone needs for sleeping at night.

Yet, as we saw, Marcos seems to believe that street people should be allowed to sleep on the sidewalks. Why? Because he views mental patients as having legitimate claims to an array of special rights, among them the right to sleep on the sidewalks. It is an absurd inference. Medical patients have a right to reject treatment. But we do not interpret the fact that arthritics have the right to reject treatment to mean that they have the right to copulate on the sidewalks. Clearly, men and women have the right to have sexual intercourse—but not anywhere: in private, yes; in public, no. The same reasoning applies to sleeping, eating, urinating, or defecating. We have a basic right to engage in these acts—but not on other people's property without their consent. The street person who disrupts the public order by sleeping on the sidewalk violates the rights of others just as surely as the person who disrupts traffic by leading a political protest without permission to do so. The argument that we should excuse a homeless person's sleeping on the sidewalk because he has no other choice and hence no criminal intent to act illegally is no more convincing than the argument that we should excuse a poor person's stealing because he has no other choice and hence no criminal intent to act illegally.

Regardless of whether mental patients are deprived of rights or given rights, the fact remains that we consider it a legitimate use of state power to incarcerate them: all we need to do is declare them "dangerous to themselves or others." Months after picking Joyce Brown off the sidewalk and taking her, against her will, to Bellevue, psychiatric and legal authorities were still deliberating what to do with her. Like medieval theologians deliberating how many angels can dance on the head of a pin, New York City's mental health experts were deliberating how much Haldol, if any, this allegedly psychotic woman needed:

> In testimony over the last two days in a courtroom at Bellevue Hospital, Dr. Maeve Mahon, the psychiatrist who had been treating Miss Brown at the hospital, said Miss Brown refused to shower regularly, sometimes talked and laughed to herself, made threatening gestures to staff members and was abusive to black men on the hospital staff. Miss Brown is black. Dr. Mahon asked the court for permission to administer

Haldol, an antipsychotic drug, over a three-week period to test whether it had a beneficial effect on Miss Brown's condition.[23]

The standard scenario then unfolded. New York Civil Liberties Union attorneys produced psychiatrists who testified that Brown was not psychotic and hence did not need Haldol. Attorneys for New York City responded "that without medication, Miss Brown would be forced to remain in the hospital without receiving any benefit from it." Naturally, the judge ordered more psychiatric examinations: "I just want a pure strain of psychiatric judgement," he said.[24] Note that every one of the players in this drama—Joyce Brown, her lawyers, the psychiatrists on both sides, the judge, the journalists—validated the fiction that although her confinement resulted in the loss of her liberty, it also provided treatment for her mental illness, and that the latter goal justifies hitting the former target.

It is bad enough that the terms *mental patient* and *right* contradict each other, just as the terms *slave* and *right* contradict each other. What makes the current debate concerning the civil rights of mental patients even more mindless are the mendacious psychiatric claims that mental illness is a condition that deprives a person of liberty, and that antipsychotic drugs are treatments that restore his lost liberty. Psychiatrists treat this falsehood as if it were fact. "Patients released from mental institutions refuse to return to inpatient care," writes the editor of a psychiatric journal.[25] Does he interpret this to mean that such patients vote with their feet, like political refugees who refuse to return to the oppressive regimes they have fled? Of course not: "[For] these misled mentally ill," he explains, "this kind of liberty, from any medical or humanistic point of view, is worse than any form of imprisonment."[26]

This comment epitomizes the psychiatrically correct thinking and speaking, and illustrates how implacably opposed psychiatrists really are to the idea that mental patients should have a right to reject treatment. Actually, psychiatrists believe that mental patients should not have any rights at all that override their (alleged) needs for psychiatric diagnosis and treatment. At a conference on involuntary hospitalization—held in New York in 1987, and sponsored by Beth Israel Medical Center—Stephen L. Rachlin, chairman of psychiatry at Nassau County Medical Center, declared: "The right to refuse treatment illustrates the clash between patients' 'rights' and their 'needs': It's one right too many."[27] Other psychiatrists agreed: "A psychiatric patient's refusal to take medication," opined a colleague, "is most often a reflection of illness, not an autonomous decision, and should be resolved on clinical, not judicial grounds."[28] Actually, neither the reasoning nor the rhetoric matters: Psychiatric tradition is enough to insure that, so far as hospitalizing and treating mental patients against their will goes, nothing really changes. Rachlin correctly concludes: "The trend to protect psychiatric patients' rights to refuse treatment by judicial review has meant little change in outcome, but greater expense, delay, and intrusion."[29]

Indeed, the courts routinely uphold the psychiatrists' recommendations. For example, in Massachusetts, "96% of patients' medication refusals were overridden by the courts."[30] The mentality of giving rights to mental patients has only added fuel to the already brightly burning fires of what I have called "therapy by the judiciary"—judges reaffirming the existence (material reality) of mental illness and its (medical) treatment by prescribing the treatment:

> One judge, having been told that Mellaril produces the least extrapyramidal side effects, ruled that all patients in such disputes be treated with Mellaril; another ordered that a patient be given Cogentin "at the first sign of any side effect." A third directed the hospital to raise a patient's dose of neuroleptic, if necessary, "but by no more than 50 mg/week."[31]

We have seen this kind of ugly foolishness happening in the past, when Religion and the State were united; and we see it happening now, when Psychiatry and the State are united. Formerly, the state validated the fiction that consecrated bread and wine were the body and blood of Jesus; now the state validates the fiction that misbehavior is a disease, and being poisoned by doctors is a treatment. The dramatic shedding of psychiatric tears over the mental patient's loss of liberty—from a "medical or humanistic point of view"—is thus worse than hypocrisy. The truth is that illness, bodily or mental, *cannot* cause loss of liberty; but that involuntary mental hospitalization is *synonymous with* the loss of such liberty.

I submit that we should not chase after every violation of the rights of mental patients. I say this not because helping a single person out of a single predicament is not a morally meritorious effort, but because a coercive-statist psychiatric system can create new abuses faster than we can abolish the old ones (assuming we can even do that). Instead, rational concern for human well-being—for sane and insane persons alike— must, as Roger Pilon observed, entail a concern about those systems that tend to the protection of human rights and those that tend to their violation. Far from trying to separate the moral from the political or economic, then, far from trying to avoid "politicizing" one's moral concern, those with a deep and abiding interest in human rights must come in the end to the realization that human rights constitutes precisely that nexus between the moral and the political and economic that theorists of the 17th and 18th centuries, theorists of the classical liberal tradition, recognized so well and articulated so clearly. They must come to realize, in short, that human rights are what political and economic systems at bottom are all about.[32]

Candor and decency require that we acknowledge that, because of its inexorable social consequences, the idea of mental illness embodies within itself the notion of diminished or absent personal autonomy. To ignore this is tantamount to engaging in double-talk. Thus, when an expert on the rights of mental patients asserts that "mentally ill persons should receive humane, dignified, and professional treatment"[33]—as does Timothy W. Harding, the leader of an expert mission of the International Commission of Jurists to investigate allegations of mistreatment of mental patients in Japan—he is, in effect, pleading for his own right to define what constitutes mental illness and its appropriate involuntarily treatment.[34] Inasmuch as the commission comes down squarely in support of psychiatric coercions when required by what mental health professionals consider to be the best interests of the patients, the central problem of so-called psychiatric abuses remains untouched: How do we make psychiatric treatment dignified when the patient rejects the psychiatrist's intrusion into his life?

Is there a way out of this labyrinth? There is for those looking for an exit. I add this caveat because, for perfectly good reasons, many persons are not looking for such an exit. Involuntary, institutional psychiatry, appropriately adapted to time and place, serves the interests of many individuals and groups: Mental health professionals like it because it legitimizes them not only as healers but as the protectors of society as well; mental patients—for the most part, most of the time—like it because it legitimizes them as sick and offers them an escape from the day-to-day cares of normal life; last but not least, the relatives of mental patients, politicians, and the legal system like it because it provides them with a legitimate mechanism for distancing themselves from mental patients and subjecting the patients to the control of the state.[35] To paraphrase Voltaire, if there were no mental illness, it would be necessary to invent it.

But it is not necessary to invent mental illness, as it has been handed down to us by our ancestors, authenticated by the most solid scientific credentials imaginable. Mental illness, we are assured, is either a proven or putative disease of the human body as a biological machine. The ultimate fallacy in this idea is that it is believed to morally justify the psychiatrist's domination of the mental patient on the one hand, and the mental patient's evasion of his responsibility to mind his own business on the other. By the latter, I mean that if mental patients are to be accorded the same rights as other adults in our society, then they must also be expected to assume the same responsibilities. In short, they must be seen as moral agents who have the duty to take care of their own biological, personal, and financial needs and the needs of those who depend on them, and to respect the rights of others and the law of the land. Accordingly, if they break the law, they must be punished in the criminal justice system, not treated in the mental health system. In proportion as we excuse persons with mental, but not with medical, illnesses, we join the chorus of hypocrites singing the theme song of the mental health industry— "Mental illness is like any other illness"—all the while making certain that the phrase, *the rights of mental patients*, continues to serve the best interests of the singers.

Curiously, my insistence that we view so-called mental patients as persons first, and as mentally ill second, has led Cambridge University professor Sir Martin Roth to pay me what I consider to be the highest compliment possible. In the final paragraph of a scathing attack on my work, Roth writes:

> He [Szasz] has been a powerful fighter for the freedoms, rights and responsibilities of psychiatric patients. The attitude of the law and the legal profession to psychiatry and mental disorder has been transformed by the writings of Thomas Szasz, in the USA. He is obsessed by the need he feels for psychiatric patients, psychotic or neurotic, to be accepted by us all as human beings of no less value than ourselves. . . . [36]

To that indictment, I proudly plead guilty. However, Roth does not stop here but adds:

> . . . and therefore not ill; for if they are thought of as mentally ill, they cannot but be devalued, dehumanized, degraded. This is the conclusion at which he has to arrive; and hence comes the necessity to stand logic on its head in order to get there. [37]

The phrase "and therefore not ill" is rubbish and has nothing to do with my insistence that we distinguish the literal meanings of disease from their metaphorical meanings. As for "standing logic on its head," the less said the better. Perhaps I should add here that while I reject the moral and political legitimacy of placing a person, with or without due process of law, in the class called "mentally ill," I accept the legitimacy of placing him, with due process of law (explicitly excluding the use of so-called psychiatric expertise from the proceedings), in the class called "incompetent."[38]

I should like to reiterate that the very idea of giving rights to the mental patient expresses, once again, society's collective contempt of him; and that the mental patient's failure to protest against this ritual reinforces society's collective sense of being justified in patronizing him. After all, Catholics do not have a specially identified right to accept or reject Holy Communion. Jews do not have a specially identified right to accept or reject the Jewish dietary laws. Patients with arthritis or diabetes do not have specially identified rights to accept or reject treatment for their diseases. Mental patients, however, are specifically granted a right to treatment and a right to reject treatment. But so long as they are denied the right to disclaim having a mental disease and reject the role of mental patient, their "psychiatric rights" are not merely worthless but an insult to their intelligence and dignity.

8

The Illusion of Drug Abuse Treatment

> Hazardous Use—*Use of a drug that will probably
> lead to harmful consequences. . . . This category
> includes the idea of risky behavior, e.g., smoking
> 1 pack of cigarettes a day.*
> —World Health Organization

Because drug abuse treatment involves not only ideas such as disease and treatment but also the power of the state, it is a politically controversial and semantically deceptive subject. As I have maintained for nearly four decades, our society habitually conflates and confuses two kinds of diseases and two kinds of treatments. The first kind of disease, exemplified by AIDS, is discovered by doctors; the second kind, exemplified by drug abuse, is mandated by legislators and decreed by judges. Similarly, the first kind of treatment, exemplified by the surgical removal of a gall bladder, is advised by doctors and authorized by competent patients; the second kind, exemplified by participation in a court-ordered drug treatment program, is imposed by judges on defendants accused or convicted of violating drug laws. I reject the scientific validity of placing rule-breaking behavior in the same category as bodily disease—and accepting both, on equal footing, as diseases; and I repudiate the moral legitimacy of equating a drug defendant's submission to a court-imposed intervention with a free adult's participation in a medical intervention—and accepting both, on equal footing, as treatments.

Moreover, not only does coercion do moral violence to the concept of treatment, but the entire drug abuse treatment enterprise rests on a pharmacologically phony foundation. If a person buys methadone on the street and takes it, he is a criminal; but if he gets methadone from a government program and takes it, he is a patient. This is a scenario fit for a humorist, a cynic, an opportunist, or an idiot—but it is not fit for a decent, educated, law-abiding citizen of a free country. If not for the hysteria of the drug war, I would think it unnecessary to point out that illegally obtained penicillin cures syphilis just as effectively as legally obtained penicillin.

At the end of this medically violent century, we ought to know better than to view the medical profession as independent of, and morally superior to, politics and the society of which it is a part. The activities of the Nazi doctors, for which many were hanged at Nuremberg, were not aberrations imposed on a holy healing profession by a totalitarian regime; on the contrary, they were the inexorable manifestations of the physician's dependence on the society he serves and of the medical profession's traditional function as, *inter alia*, an instrument of social control. Without belaboring this painful subject, suffice it to say here that physicians assisted the Inquisition; supported, in peace as well as war, the military efforts of all nations; and regularly serve, in all modern societies, as an extralegal police force to control deviance—especially through involuntary psychiatric interventions. The medical profession's present support of the War on Drugs is thus just one more episode in its long history of participation in religious, national, and political conflicts.

The plain and simple fact is that American law, medicine, and public opinion now regard not only involuntary confinement in a mental hospital, but also involuntary participation in a so-called drug treatment program as a bona fide medical treatment. The following statement, in the *Handbook of Drug Control in the United States*, edited by University of Delaware Professor James Inciardi and U.S. Senator Joseph Biden, Jr. (D-Del.), is illustrative: "Civil commitment is frequently used with addicts who are arrested for criminal activity; with criminal charges pending, the addict can be coerced into treatment and retained long enough to receive the benefits of a treatment program."[1] I venture to say that the most important function of our fashionable drug treatment rhetoric is to distract us from the fact that the drug user wants the drug of his choice, not the drug treatment the authorities impose on him. We are flooded with news stories about addicts robbing people to get money to pay for drugs. But has anyone ever heard of an addict robbing a person to get money to pay for drug treatment?

Thus, if we were to view the whole package of criminalized drug use plus legalized coercion masquerading as "drug treatment" from a free market perspective, we would see the drug user's behavior as his existential and economic demand for the drug of his choice; and we would see the drug prohibitionist's so-called services as deceptive and coercive meddling deliberately mislabeled as "therapy." Indeed, so long as the drug counselor (or whatever he is called) acts as a paid agent of the state (or some other third party in conflict with the self-defined interests of the drug user), we would have to define his intervention as interference not only in the life of his nominal client but in the free market in drugs as well. Frederic Bastiat (1801–1850), the French political-economic thinker and pioneer free-marketeer, warned against all this, and more. "To rob the public," he observed, "it is necessary to deceive it. To deceive it is to persuade it that it is being robbed for its own benefit, and to induce it to accept, in exchange for its property, services that are fictitious or often even worse."[2]

If ever there were services that are "fictitious or even worse," they are our current publicly financed drug treatment services. The wisdom of our language reveals the truth and supports the cogency of these reflections. We do not call convicts "consumers of prison services," or conscripts "consumers of military services"; but we call committed mental patients "consumers of mental health services" and paroled addicts "consumers of drug treatment services." We might as well call drug traffickers, conscripted by ex-czar William Bennett for beheading, "consumers of Guillotine services." After all, Dr. Guillotine was a doctor, and Mr. Bennett used to teach ethics.

To be sure, persons drafted as convicts, conscripts, and "chemically dependent persons" all receive certain services, such as food, shelter, clothing, and antidrug propaganda. The provision of such services is then used to mask the fact that the beneficiaries would prefer that their benefactors left them alone. Like the mythologizing of personal problems as mental *diseases*, so the mythologizing of illegal drug use as a *disease* has been overwhelmingly successful: In 1991, the federal government spent more than $1 billion on *drug treatment research*. Enthusiasm for such "research" is not diminished by the fact that, according to a General Accounting Office report released in September 1990, "researchers know little more about the best way to treat various drug addictions than they did 10 years ago."[3]

With the intensification of the War on Drugs, manifested by the addition of drug treatment to the warriors' arsenal of drug punishment, the American people are not only being criminalized by a drug-police state, they are also being robbed by it. Asked by *Psychiatric Times* what he considers "to be the major accomplishments of the federal government's [drug] program," Herbert D. Kleber, M.D., professor of psychiatry at Yale and deputy director of the Office of National Drug Control Policy, replied:

> When President Bush took office, the federal budget [for drug control] was $5.5 billion; it is now in excess of $11 billion. . . . The federal treatment budget, for example, has been increased from $850 million to more than $1.6 billion over the past three years. . . . In the past few years, we have increased the [drug abuse] treatment budget for the Bureau of Prisons from $2 million to $22 million.[4]

When the reporter asked Kleber if "there is any indication that any of the pharmacologic treatments for drug abuse are particularly effective" he replied: "There is no hard evidence yet, but there are some promising leads."[5]

It is difficult to treat a disease that exists. It is easier to treat one that does not: All that is needed is control of the patient's liberty, the taxpayer's money, and the medical vocabulary.

9

The Case Against Suicide Prevention

The preventive function of government, however, is far more liable to be abused, to the prejudice of liberty, than the punitory function; for there is hardly any part of the legitimate freedom of action of a human being which would not admit of being represented, and fairly too, as increasing the facilities for some form or other of delinquency.

—John Stuart Mill, *On Liberty*

My aim in this essay is to rebut the contemporary view that suicide is a mental health problem, that psychiatric practitioners and institutions have a professional duty to try to prevent it, and that it is a legitimate function of the state to empower such professionals and institutions—especially psychiatrists and mental hospitals—to impose coercive interventions on persons diagnosed as posing a suicidal risk. Because of these assumptions, should a person formally identified as a patient kill himself while in the care of a mental health clinician or clinic, the latter is likely to be sued for, and may be found guilty of, professional negligence for failing to prevent his suicide.

I reject this perspective and offer, instead, another view of suicide—as that of an act by a moral agent, for which that agent himself is ultimately responsible. Rejecting suicide prevention in principle, and eschewing it as a professional practice, would protect the mental health clinician from having to play self-contradictory roles; would protect the mental health client from having to submit to coercion in the name of suicide prevention; and would protect the American people from having to pay for a so-called health policy that undermines the ethic of self-responsibility on which our nation ostensibly rests.

147

I want to emphasize, at the outset, that I am opposed only to coercive methods of preventing, or trying to prevent, suicide. However, it would be mendacious to deny that, in practice, suicide prevention rests on the use of force, or on the threat of its use, to restrain the would-be suicide. Indeed, the term *prevention*, bracketed with the term *suicide*, implies coercion. Preventive medical measures, exemplified by vaccinating children against contagious diseases, are typically (although not always) backed by the force of the law. In contrast, advice, guidance, or instruction regarding pregnancy or marriage are called abortion and marriage "counseling." It would be awkward, and wrong, to call such counseling "abortion prevention," "marriage prevention," or "divorce prevention."

Psychiatrists (and other mental health professionals) bear an especially heavy burden of responsibility with respect to the moral dilemmas posed by suicide; hence, they must be especially thoughtful and forthright about where they come down on the issue of coercive suicide prevention. Just as mental health professionals reject—as ethically and professionally unacceptable—sexual relations between therapists and clients, so they could also reject—as ethically and professionally unacceptable—coercing clients who they think or fear might kill themselves. Alternatively, mental health professionals could individually choose to accept or reject coercive suicide prevention as a part of the service they render—each practitioner clearly identified to the public by his stance toward this practice. Anyone identified as a therapist or member of a helping profession could thus elect to embrace coercive suicide prevention, as the psychiatrist—qua life-saving clinician in the hospital—typically does, and is expected to do by custom and law; or he could eschew such coercion, as the priest—qua soul-saving cleric in the confessional—does, and is required to do by custom, religion, and law. Opting for either course would be defensible and moral. But, given the dilemmas posed by suicide and suicide prevention, trying to play both roles at once and claiming to serve the best interests of both the individual and society, is impossible to achieve and immoral to attempt.

Failure to prevent suicide is now one of the leading reasons for successful malpractice suits against psychiatrists and psychiatric institutions. This situation is the inevitable consequence of the way suicide is now viewed by mental health professionals, lawyers, judges, and other educated persons.

Because the result of suicide is death, it is not surprising that people want to hold someone or something responsible for it. In the history of Western civilization, the eighteenth century marks a dramatic change in the perception of suicide. Prior to that time, suicide was considered to be both a sin and a crime for which the actor was responsible; since then, suicide has increasingly been regarded as a manifestation of madness for which the actor is not responsible.[1] Thus, long before suicide was decriminalized, the responsibility of the self-murderer for his deed was annulled by declaring him, posthumously, *non compos mentis*, a tactic whose dangerous moral and political implications did not go unnoticed. In 1755, William Blackstone sounded this warning against the practice:

> But this excuse [of lunacy] ought not to be strained to the length to which our coroner's juries are apt to carry it, viz., that every act of suicide is an evidence of insanity; as if every man who acts contrary to reason had no reason at all; for the same argument would prove every other criminal *non compos*, as well as the self-murderer.[2]

Although Blackstone foresaw this "abuse" of the idea of insanity, it is precisely the elastic and strategic character of the concept that makes it so attractive to the modern mind.[3]

However, the history of suicide is not germane to our present concerns. Suffice it to mention here that the view of suicide as self-murder originates from the Judeo-Christian cosmology in which God is viewed as both giving and taking each human being's life. Taking one's own life is thus a grievous offense against God. The modern, scientistic view of suicide represents a secularized version of the same belief. "We are now in agreement," declared Stanley Yolles, former director of the National Institute of Mental Health, "that this [suicide] is a public health matter and that the state should combat the disease of suicide."[4] The idea that anyone who kills himself is crazy exonerates the suicide from wrongdoing, but stigmatizes the act as a symptom of insanity.

The psychiatrically popularized image of suicide today—as a mental abnormality or illness, or a symptom of such a condition—explains why mental health professionals, philosophers, and ethicists, as well as lay persons, are all so skittish about suicide that it is virtually impossible to engage in a reasoned examination of this subject. Why is suicide considered to be a priori bad or undesirable? And, if it is considered bad because it injures society, then why is it not treated as a crime, as it used to be, and punished by the state? Or, if it is considered bad because it injures the victim's soul, then why is it not treated as a sin , as it used to be, and punished by the Church? (Persons who kill themselves are no longer denied a Christian or Jewish burial.) Finally, if suicide is considered bad because it injures both the suicide and others, like a disease (as people now seem to believe), then why is it not treated by specialists who know how to treat "it"? But who knows how to "treat" suicide? No one.

Instead of seriously pondering such questions, people now prefer to explain away the problem of suicide by claiming to view it scientifically, creating an image of it that combines the features not only of sin, sickness, and crime, but also of irrationality, incompetence, and insanity. The result is a stubborn unwillingness to view suicide as we view other morally freighted acts—like abortion or divorce—as good or bad, desirable or undesirable, depending on the circumstances in which the act occurs and the criteria by which it is judged.

If a person suffers harm that he attributes to his relationship with a professional, it does not automatically follow that the professional is guilty of negligence (malpractice). To successfully prosecute a suit for professional negligence, the plaintiff must show that the professional had a specific duty to perform—typically, because he voluntarily assumed said duty; that he performed his duty negligently or not at all; that the plaintiff suffered injuries as a result; and that the injury is directly attributable to the malperformance or nonperformance of the professional's duty.[5]

What constitutes a professional's duty? *Black's Law Dictionary* states: "As a technical term of the law, 'duty' signifies . . . that which a person owes to another. An obligation to do a thing."[6] How does a person or party incur such an obligation? Typically, by contracting for it—for example, as an airline company does when it promises, in exchange for a sum of money, to transport a passenger from place A to place B, and to do so without causing injury to the passenger during the flight.

The main reason mental health professionals and mental institutions are often found liable for a patient's suicide is because they assume the duty (responsibility) of preventing suicide. It is important to emphasize that, as a rule, in our society, people are free to seek or not seek professional help, and professionals are free to assume or not assume a particular duty. For example, a Catholic gynecologist, determined to abide by the dictates of faith, is free to refuse to perform an abortion; a neurosurgeon, burdened by astronomical malpractice insurance premiums, is free to refuse to perform surgery (and limit his practice to neurology); and a mental health professional is (presumably) free, if he so chooses, to refrain from assuming the duty of trying to prevent a patient's suicide. Of course, it must be clear to the client and society alike what duties a professional assumes and declines. Mental health professionals and institutions would probably be much better protected against successful suits for failing to prevent suicide if they explicitly eschewed assuming the duty of suicide prevention as a professional service. However, as long as mental health professionals insist on imposing their services on unwilling recipients by claiming that the patients are "dangerous to themselves," they should not be surprised that when a patient commits suicide (or otherwise injures himself while under professional care), his family holds the mental health professionals responsible for failing to fulfill their promises, and that juries and courts find them guilty of professional negligence. The fact that suicide prevention—with or without the cooperation of patients—is one of the duties and services now specifically attributed to, accepted by, and expected from mental health professionals and institutions constitutes the context for my following remarks.

If a troubled individual confides his so-called suicidal ideation to a priest, the priest is not expected to intervene coercively to prevent his suicide. Neither is the lawyer who, especially if engaged in matrimonial disputes, often hears clients say such things as, "If my husband leaves me, I will kill myself." However, the mental health professional is expected to prevent suicide. If he is a psychiatrist, he has a duty to commit the patient; if he is a psychologist, social worker, nurse practitioner, or lay therapist—who is not (or not yet) licensed by the state to commit— then he is expected to make an appropriate referral to a physician (who may or may not be a psychiatrist) to forcibly prevent the patient's suicide. Although mental health professionals sometimes complain about the burden this duty entails, in the main they clearly enjoy the power and prestige that go along with it. After all, if psychiatrists did not want to engage in coercive suicide prevention, they could say so and could refuse to participate in such work. Similarly, if psychologists viewed coercive suicide prevention negatively, they too could say so, instead of seeking (as many do) the professional privilege and legal authority to involuntarily confine persons deemed to be dangerous to themselves.

Why do psychiatrists (and other mental health professionals) seek and receive special privileges and powers to intervene in the lives of so-called suicidal persons? Because in the modern view, the person who threatens to commit suicide or actually does so is typically considered to be mentally ill.[7] I need not belabor the contention that this is an absurd, parochial view of what may well be life's oldest existential option and greatest moral challenge. There is, of course, not a shred of historical, philosophical, or medical support for viewing suicide as different, in principle, from other acts or important decisions, such as getting married or divorced or having a child.

The phrase *suicide prevention* is itself a misleading slogan characteristic of our therapeutic age. Insofar as suicide is a physical possibility, there can be no suicide prevention. Insofar as suicide is a fundamental right, there ought to be no coercive suicide prevention measures or programs. If one person is to prevent another person from killing himself, the former obviously cannot, and should not be expected to, accomplish that task unless he can exercise complete control over the suicidal person. But it is either impossible to do this, or would require reducing the subject to a social status beneath that of a slave. The slave is compelled only to labor against his will; whereas the person forcibly prevented from killing himself is compelled to live against his will.

None of this means that an individual troubled by suicidal ideas or impulses should be denied the assistance he seeks, provided he can find others willing to render such assistance. It means only that expressions of so-called suicidal behavior—in any of their now-familiar psychopathological forms or shapes, such as suicidal ideation, suicidal impulse, suicide attempt, and so forth—would no longer qualify as a justification for coercing the subject. Were such a policy adopted, people would have to make do with noncoercive methods of preventing suicide, just as they must now make do with noncoercive methods of preventing other forms of self-harming actions, such as warnings on packages of cigarettes or on bottles of beer.

No one can deny that policies aimed at preventing suicide by means of legal and psychiatric coercion imply a paternalistic attitude toward the patient, and require giving certain privileges and powers to a special class of protectors vis-à-vis a special class of victims. All such solutions for human problems are purchased at the cost of creating the classic problem of "Who shall guard the guardians?" The demonstrable harms generated by the mistakes and misuses of the powers of mental health professionals and judges (delegated to them on the ground that they are protecting suicidal persons from themselves) must be balanced against the alleged or ostensible benefits generated by coercive policies of suicide prevention. Since we have no generally agreed upon criteria for adjudicating controversies concerning such a trade-off, our acceptance or rejection of coercive suicide prevention is best viewed as a manifestation of our moral principles and psychiatric premises—especially about free will and personal responsibility on the one hand, and mental illness and therapeutic paternalism on the other hand.

Ironically, psychiatrists now stigmatize and punish the threat of suicide in much the same way as priests used to stigmatize and punish the act—but with one important difference: The theory and practice of coercive suicide prevention also stigmatizes the psychiatrists. To start with, concepts such as "suicidal risk" and "suicidal danger" are ambiguous terms that cover a wide variety of situations— from persons who actually threaten to kill themselves (and may or may not mean to do so), to persons who explicitly deny any desire to commit suicide (though they may or may not plan to do so) but whose relatives or psychiatrists fear they might kill themselves. By incarcerating and involuntarily "treating" such persons, psychiatrists patronize their patients and promise them and society more than they can deliver, doubly compromising their integrity. In an effort to prevent suicide by force, psychiatrists necessarily ally themselves with the police powers of the state, thus defining themselves as foes rather than friends of individual liberty and responsibility. Moreover, it requires no special psychological perspicacity to entertain the possibility that attempts to prevent suicide may instead abet and encourage it, as Antonin Artaud so eloquently argued:

> It was in fact, after a conversation with Dr. Gachet that van Gogh, as if nothing were the matter, went back to his room and killed himself. I myself spent nine years in an insane asylum and I never had the obsession of suicide, but I know that each conversation with a psychiatrist, every morning at the time of his visit, made me want to hang myself, realizing that I would not be able to cut his throat.[8]

We are ready now to consider the question of the mental health professional's responsibility for the suicide of a client or patient. First, we must clarify what we mean when we speak of one person's responsibility toward another, especially of a professional person's responsibility toward a client. We use the term *responsible* to describe a person's accountability for the conduct or welfare of himself or others. For example, competent adults are responsible for themselves, and, as parents, they are responsible for their children.

The idea of responsibility is intertwined with two other concepts: liberty and control. Liberty and responsibility are, in fact, two sides of the same coin. Ordinarily, we assume that adults are moral agents endowed with free will: That is, they choose their behavior from among a range of options. Hence, they are responsible for their actions: We praise or blame them, depending on whether we judge their conduct to be good or bad.

Where there is no freedom, there is no responsibility: We do not hold infants responsible for their behavior; duress is a complete excuse in the criminal law; and so forth. And where there is no control, there can be no responsibility: A person cannot be held responsible for something he does not control. Asserting that "John is responsible for James" (for his welfare, health, not committing suicide, and so on) is tantamount to asserting that John can, and indeed must, have enough control over James to bring about or maintain the condition specified for James. This is why persons who want to assume control over others typically claim to be responsible for them (called "paternalism"), and why persons who want to reject responsibility for their own conduct typically claim to have no control over their actions (called "mental illness").

The foregoing principles are recognized in contractual arrangements—for example, when a bank trustee is empowered to manage someone else's money, or an anesthesiologist is empowered to put someone else to sleep. Such experts undertake to exercise a specific responsibility, for the proper discharge of which they are granted control over specific objects or functions (the client's money, the patient's respiration). In every such situation, the controllers become responsible for what they control, and *only* for what they control. It follows, then, that anyone who assumes the task of preventing another person from committing suicide must assume the most far-reaching control over that person's capacity to act. Because it is virtually impossible to prevent the suicide of a person determined to kill himself, and because forcibly imposed interventions to prevent suicide deprive the patient of liberty and dignity, the use of psychiatric coercion to prevent suicide is at once impractical and immoral. Of course, because children have neither the rights nor the responsibilities of adults; and because, unlike adults, children are typically treated coercively by the medical system (as well as in other situations)—we must carefully distinguish between policies aimed at children and policies aimed at adults. The principle of coercive paternalism obliterates this basic distinction. In this discussion, I am concerned only with *adult* suicidal persons, and only with those subjected to *involuntary* interventions (mental health interventions provided non-coercively for voluntary clients pose no special conceptual or moral problems).

What, then, *is*, and what *should be*, the mental health professional's responsibility, insofar as he deals with a suicidal patient? My reply to the first question is that the clinician's responsibility vis-à-vis such a patient is whatever the law says it is. As for what the clinician's responsibility vis-à-vis the suicidal patient should be, my answer is that it should be similar to that of any other health professional's vis-à-vis his competent, adult patient. If the patient seeks help for being suicidal, the mental health professional has a moral obligation—and, depending on the circumstances, perhaps also a legal obligation—to provide some sort of help for him. However, if the patient does not want such help and actively rejects it, then the mental health professional's duty ought to be to leave him alone (or, perhaps, to try to persuade him to accept some sort of help).

In short, I object to our present policies of suicide prevention because they downgrade the responsibility of the individual (called a "patient," even if he explicitly rejects that role) for the conduct of his own life and death. Because I value individual liberty highly and am convinced that liberty and responsibility are indivisible, I want to enlarge the scope of liberty and responsibility. In the present instance, this means opposing policies of suicide prevention that minimize the responsibility of individuals for killing themselves, and supporting policies that maximize their responsibility for doing so. I believe we should make it more difficult for the suicidal person to *reject responsibility for killing himself*, and for the mental health professional to *assume responsibility for keeping such a person alive*. To achieve this goal, we would have to hold every adult responsible for his behavior and, perhaps temporarily, make use of a psychiatric will.[9]

In a free society a person is not only presumed to be innocent until proven guilty, but also presumed sane and responsible until proven insane and irresponsible. This important principle is now being eroded, due in no small part to the ideology of mental illness and the activities of mental health professionals. For example, many adult, mentally competent

Americans now claim that they are not responsible for having smoked cigarettes and mental health professionals eagerly support their claim with expert testimony in suits against tobacco companies.[10] The belief that we can have liberty without responsibility is, of course, an illusion people are often unwilling to relinquish until it is too late to do so.

The presumption of sanity, like the presumption of innocence, has far-reaching implications, especially insofar as a person's right to his own body is concerned.[11] Consider, for example, our contemporary attitude toward procreation. Whether a person creates another human life is now almost completely separated from nature. Contraception and abortion are legal and widely practiced, and we have access to sophisticated techniques of artificial fertilization and permissive rules for surrogate motherhood. The decision to create or not create new life has thus been rendered largely independent of both biological and social constraints (such as marriage or the ability or willingness to support a child) and, like never before in history, is (potentially) a matter of personal choice and individual responsibility. Notwithstanding such considerations, as well as the far-reaching social consequences of procreation, we treat creating a child as if it were an inalienable right.

I cite these familiar facts to draw a parallel between procreation and suicide: The former consists of multiplying one's life, the other of nullifying it. Both decisions have a profound impact, for good or ill, on the actors, their families, and the society of which they are a part. In the case of procreation, we recognize the moral complexity of the phenomenon—specifically, that every baby's life is infinitely precious, but that irresponsible procreation is dangerous, destructive of the welfare of both the infant and society. Nevertheless, we in the West impose no coercive measures on persons innocent of crime (not even on minors) to prevent procreation—as if procreation were never undesirable enough to warrant such preventive measures.

In the case of suicide, however, we distort and deny the moral complexity of the phenomenon—specifically, that although life is precious, disease, disability, and dishonor may render a person's life not worth living and may thus make suicide a blessing for the subject, his family, and society. Moreover, we (in the West) impose far-reaching measures of coercion on every would-be suicide, even the hopelessly sick and the very old—as if suicide were never desirable enough to justify permitting it.[12]

Such reflections incline me to believe that it would be morally and politically desirable to accord suicide the status of a basic human right (in its strict, political-philosophical sense). When I say this, I emphatically do not mean that killing oneself is, ipso facto, good or praiseworthy (a disclaimer I emphasize only because the meaning of the word *right* is now often so misinterpreted). I mean only that the power of the state should not be legitimately deployed to prohibit or prevent persons from killing themselves. The point is simple but often forgotten: For example, when we say that freedom of religion is a right, we do not mean that we must accept all religions as equally ethical or fit for modern life; we mean only that we ought to abstain from deploying the power of the state to promote the religion we like, and prohibit those we dislike.

Actually, the distinction between the illegal and the immoral is deeply ingrained in Anglo-American law. Thus, certain acts are regarded not only as crimes but also as violations of widely shared moral values: for example, the unprovoked killing of another person is a *malum in se*, a wrong in itself. Certain other acts are regarded as crimes only because they violate existing laws without being immoral: for example, a parking violation is a *malum prohibitum*, a wrong because it is prohibited. Finally, there are acts some people regard as wrongs to be prohibited by law, but others do not: for example, Jim Crow laws or drug laws. In a free, secular society, such prohibitions ought to be illegal, because the behaviors they seek to control deprive no one of life, liberty, or property; they merely offend the values of a particular caste or creed.

The effort to seriously ponder the issue of suicide probes some of our most passionately held, but not universally shared, beliefs about ending our own lives. Is killing oneself like homicide, and hence properly called "suicide?" Or is it more like birth control, and better termed "death control"? As polls and other evidence clearly show, Americans view suicide ambivalently, as both a dreaded enemy and a trusted friend.

The belief that it is the legitimate function of the state to coerce persons because they might kill themselves is a characteristically modern, quasi-therapeutic idea, catering at once to our craving for dependency and omnipotence. The result is an intricate web of interventions and institutions that have themselves become powerful engines of hypocrisy and seemingly indispensable mechanisms for satisfying human needs now buried in hidden agendas.

It has taken a long time to get mental health professionals deeply enmeshed in the suicide business, and it will take a long time to get them out of it. In the meantime, mental health professionals and their clients are doomed to wander aimlessly in the existential-legal labyrinth generated by treating suicide as if it constituted a mental health problem. However, if we refuse to play a part in the drama of coercive suicide prevention, then we shall be sorely tempted to conclude that mental health professionals and their partners in suicide richly deserve each other and the torment each is so ready and eager to inflict on the other.

10

The Psychiatric Will

*Nobody may compel me to be happy in his own
way. Paternalism is the greatest despotism imaginable.*

—Immanuel Kant

The psychiatric examination, diagnosis, treatment, and hospitalization
of persons against their will—in and out of psychiatric, medical, and
other institutions—form a rich web of social policies legitimized by
tradition, sanctioned by science, and articulated by law. Although ideas
have practical consequences, and although social policies usually rest on
and are justified by ideas, the fact remains that ideas can be fully effective
only against other ideas. To put it differently, arguments can be used only
to rebut other arguments; they cannot be used, at least not directly, to
change social policies or legal practices. Witch-hunts and the enslave-
ment of blacks in the United States spring to mind as obvious examples.
Although many people believed, and some even argued, that witches did
not exist and that blacks were persons, witch-hunting did not stop until
the witch craze had run its course, and slavery did not end in the United
States until the South had been defeated in a brutal war by the North. It
seems unlikely, then, that ideas and arguments alone will prevail against
the well-established practices of coercive psychiatry either.

This conclusion should not strike us as particularly surprising or
pessimistic. It is a simple fact of life that just as individuals cannot be
talked out of personal habits sanctioned by their conscience, so people
cannot be talked out of collective practices sanctioned by their historical
tradition and law. In each case, whether it be personal conduct or social
custom, one pattern of behavior must be replaced by another. In this
chapter, my aim is to propose a new social policy that respects and
protects equally the ideas and interests of both the proponents and the
opponents of involuntary psychiatric interventions.

159

First, I shall briefly restate the traditional justifications for involuntary mental hospitalization and treatment and my previous arguments against such interventions. Then, I shall add a fresh—and, it seems to me, irrefutable—argument to the case against commitment practices, cast in the form of a new legal mechanism that accommodates the legitimate interests and demands of both the psychiatric protectionists and the psychiatric voluntarists.

A brief remark about terminology is in order here. In my earlier writings, using the analogy with involuntary servitude, I used the term *psychiatric abolitionist* to refer to the person who wants to abolish involuntary psychiatry.[1] Respecting the self-declared motives of both parties to the conflict, I here use the term *psychiatric protectionist*, to refer to the person who—to protect the psychotic patient from the consequences of his illness—supports the use of involuntary psychiatric interventions; and I use the term *psychiatric voluntarist*, to refer to the person who—to protect individuals from the consequences of psychiatric coercion—supports the use of voluntary psychiatric interactions only. Enlisting the power of the state to prohibit psychiatric relations between consenting adults is, of course, just as inimical to the spirit of liberty as is enlisting it to impose psychiatric relations on unwilling patients. The policy I propose attains the libertarian goal of protection from coerced psychiatry without, at the same time, depriving persons—who wish to be the beneficiaries of coerced psychiatric protections—from access to involuntary psychiatric interventions.

The justifications for psychiatric coercions, enshrined in the history and vocabulary of psychiatry as well as in the terminology of commitment statutes throughout the world, fall into three distinct categories.

The first centers on the conjoint concepts of mental illness and mental treatment. It is believed that just as some persons suffer from bodily diseases, so others suffer from mental diseases, and that these diseases, too, are, more or less, amenable to medical treatment. Mental patients are thus urged to submit to psychiatric treatment—voluntarily. However, since mental illness is believed to impair the judgment of those who suffer from it, it is held that some mental patients who "need treatment" do not avail themselves of it because they lack insight into their condition— hence, treatment must be imposed on them against their will. The following is a typical statement of this view: "The nature of many psychiatric illnesses is such that the denial of a need for treatment is an inherent element of the disease itself."[2] Ostensibly, this claim establishes both the need and the justification for hospitalizing and treating against their will persons afflicted with mental diseases. I object to this argument because I hold that mental illness is a metaphor —a label we attach to certain unwanted behaviors. Since there are no mental diseases, there can be no treatments for them.[3]

The second justification for commitment is "dangerousness to one-self"—a phrase that ostensibly denotes the presence of an alleged condition, called "mental illness," which people "have," and that makes them starve, mutilate, and kill themselves. The policy of commitment, or involuntary mental hospitalization—based on the principle of *parens patriae*—is then invoked to deal with the threat to the patient's health and life, and with the havoc his behavior is likely to create in the family or among the people who are forced to witness his behavior. A respected defender of psychiatric coercion puts this argument as follows: "It must be acknowledged that these severely ill people are not capable at a conscious level of deciding what is best for themselves, and that in order to help them examine their behavior and motivation, it is necessary that they be alive and available for treatment."[4] My disagreement with this view rests on the premise that in a free society bodily and personal self-ownership is a basic human right; that it is impossible to draw a satisfactory line of demarcation between self-injurious behavior due to mental illness and self-injurious behavior not due to mental illness; and that those who wish to help troubled and troubling persons called "mental patients" should be satisfied with offering help to their would-be clients and should be prevented by law from imposing help on them by force.[5]

The third justification for commitment, invoked with increasing fervor and frequency, is "dangerousness to others."[6] This justification rearticulates the ancient idea that the insane person is "mad"—that, like a "wild beast," he is dangerous to society and hence a fit subject for forcible confinement and segregation. This idea was forcefully rearticulated by the Supreme Court in its celebrated *Donaldson* decision. "A State," ruled the Court, "cannot constitutionally confine without more [treatment] a *nondangerous* individual."[7] I object to this argument because I believe that it is the duty of the state to prosecute and punish persons who deprive others of life, liberty, or property, and to leave those who commit no such offenses alone. The right to self-ownership implies that dangerousness to self is a right as well; and that (certain kinds) of dangerousness to others is a crime that the state must control by means of the criminal law.

The differences between the psychiatric protectionist and the psychiatric voluntarist are rooted in the different views each has of the world about him—a difference dramatically displayed in the danger each fears, and from which each seeks protection by means of appropriate policies: The psychiatric protectionist fears psychosis and the dire consequences of psychiatric neglect; whereas the psychiatric voluntarist fears forced psychiatric confinement and the dire consequences of compulsory psychiatric treatment.

Clearly, the proponents and opponents of involuntary psychiatric interventions reached an impasse long ago. Instead of recognizing and acknowledging that this impasse is rooted in the antagonists' different philosophical, political, and psychiatric premises, the patient-rights activists and the psychiatrists have turned to the courts to resolve the conflicts between them. But judges can resolve these conflicts no better than legislators or psychiatrists could resolve them. Conflicts of self-interest, differences in our values and perception of the world about us and our place in it, and, last but not least, imbalances of raw power cannot be recognized, much less reconciled, so long as they are concealed by the "psychotic" claims of patients, the "therapeutic" claims of psychiatrists, and the "judicial" claims of judges. The courts can give us "therapy by the judiciary," but they cannot give us a cognitive grasp—transcending the paralyzing presumptions of psychiatry—of the problem of which they themselves are an important part. Recent court decisions concerning patients' rights illustrate the way the courts are compounding the mischief brought before them by involuntary mental patients and institutional psychiatrists.

In a precedent-setting class-action suit in Massachusetts, the courts were asked to decide whether a committed mental patient had a right to refuse being medicated against his will.[8] The Judge, Joseph Tauro, ruled that the patients had such a right and justified his decision as follows:

> Whatever powers the Constitution has granted our government, involuntary mind control is not one of them. . . . The fact that mind control takes place in a mental institution in the form of medically sound treatment of mental disease [does not warrant] an unsanctioned intrusion on the integrity of a human being.[9]

Judge Tauro's ruling implicitly affirmed an internally contradictory proposition: namely, that some individuals are so seriously mentally ill, or are so incompetent, that it is justifiable to confine (hospitalize) them against their will; but that, nevertheless, they are mentally healthy enough, or competent enough, to refuse being drugged (treated) against their will. Although Judge Tauro's reasoning is saturated with psychiatric presumptions, his decision evoked an indignant editorial response in the *American Journal of Psychiatry*. This response illustrates how hopelessly bogged down the debate about "psychiatric rights" has become. Citing the passage quoted above, the editorial writer thundered:

> This excerpt clearly illustrates the failure of the legal mind to grasp clinical realities. The clinician would, of course, point out that a psychosis is *itself* involuntary mind control of the most extensive kind and itself represents the most severe "intrusion on the integrity of the human being." The physician seeks to liberate the patient from the chains of illness; the judge, from the chains of treatment.[10]

With nearly everyone committed to "liberating" the involuntary mental patient, and with hardly anyone interested in leaving him alone to be both free and responsible, it is small wonder that he remains infantilized and institutionalized as a ward of the judge and the psychiatrist—the role into which he was cast a very long time ago. What makes the involuntarily hospitalized mental patient's present situation different from what it has been until recently? The answer is that, in the past, psychiatrists acknowledged that psychiatric confinement entailed depriving patients of their freedom—whereas now they claim that such confinement serves only to enable them to achieve "true freedom." A report in *Psychiatric News* explained this view—which its advocates call "commitment to freedom"—as follows: "Some psychiatrists are [now] thinking not in terms of physical restrictions on freedom but of the shackles of illness itself and the patients' right to freedom from this mental restraint."[11] At the 1980 annual meeting of the American Academy of Psychiatry and Law, two prominent psychiatrists from Washington, D.C.'s Saint Elizabeth's Hospital explained this view as follows:

> Is a stuporous catatonic freer successfully refusing fluphenazine, or is his life freer if given the fluphenazine involuntarily? . . . We would submit that commitment can be justified on the grounds of enhancing the individual's future freedom. If society insisted that freedom be the only purpose of commitment, commitment to achieve a real lack of unnecessary constraints from mental illness and to increase a patient's options could be justified. . . . For a very small percentage of the mentally ill, the greatest freedom available is a community composed of specialists in dealing with the mentally ill, i.e., an asylum.[12]

These psychiatrists are clearly untroubled by the contradiction inherent in depriving a person of liberty in order, ostensibly, to liberate him; indeed, they are also untroubled about describing a mental patient as "a stuporous catatonic," while attributing to him the capacity for "successfully refusing" psychiatric medication. Through these psychiatrically colored glasses, "such an approach . . . would place psychiatry fully behind the *principle that psychiatric institutions be utilized for increasing the freedom of the mentally ill.*"[13]

Clearly, the proponents and opponents of involuntary psychiatric interventions not only disagree about the desirability of such measures, they no longer even speak the same language. With seemingly no way out of the dilemma, the disagreement between the contestants is now resolved the way such conflicts typically are—by the more powerful party using the state to impose its will on its adversary. With power in the hands of the psychiatric protectionists, psychiatric protectionism rules. Although it is unlikely that, in the foreseeable future, psychiatric abolitionists could impose their will on their adversaries, let us assume that it could happen. Would imposing psychiatric abolitionism on those who believe in mental illness and endorse involuntary psychiatric interventions be any more fair or just than the present imposition of coercive psychiatry on those who reject its premises and abhor its practices? I believe it would be—because our rights to life and liberty are so basic that we cannot contract them away: We cannot hire a person to kill us, because the state gives him no right to do so (the state allows us to kill another only in self-defense, while serving as a soldier in wartime, or as an executioner); similarly, we cannot—and should not be allowed to— hire a person to enslave us, because no private individual has the right to deprive another of liberty (only persons qua judges, members of a jury, and jailers have that right).

Above and beyond the usual justifications for commitment—such as mental illness and dangerousness to self or others—there looms an imagery about insanity that strongly supports the seeming necessity for involuntary mental hospitalization. I would summarize this imagery, which has been adroitly exploited by its advocates, as follows.

Mental illness is an illness like any other—but not quite. Ordinary medical diseases do not impair judgment or the competence to assume or reject the patient role. For example, unless he is unconscious, the patient with coronary heart disease or cancer of the colon remains in possession of his mental faculties. But serious mental diseases, so this argument runs, do impair, or even annul, the patient's judgment and competence. Viewed through psychiatric lenses, then, although the mentally ill person is seemingly conscious, he is perceived as if he were not. This justifies treating him on the model of the unconscious patient or child—not only without his consent, but even against his explicit objections.

In the countless debates about commitment in which I have engaged, especially in public forums, I have found that the proponents of involuntary psychiatric interventions frequently fall back on this imagery. Typically, the argument, framed as a personal affirmation, goes like this: "If I were to become acutely psychotic, I would hope that a psychiatrist would take care of me and treat me—without my consent, even against my will—with X, Y, or Z method, as my condition warranted." The advocate of psychiatric coercion then adduces anecdotes about involuntarily treated mental patients expressing gratitude to their psychiatrists for having saved them from the dire consequences of their psychotic illness.

Pitted against my ostensible denial of mental illness and my alleged desire to "withhold" effective treatment from persons afflicted with life-threatening mental diseases, this argument strikes many people as morally compassionate as well as medically sound. I shall try to refute it—or, perhaps more precisely, to transcend it—by proposing a fresh social policy for resolving the dilemma about commitment. However, before I do so, I want to note that a psychiatrist's personal affirmation—to the effect that, should he become psychotic, he wants to be attended by a psychiatrist and, if need be, hospitalized and treated against his will—carries no more weight than does a religious person's affirmation that, should death be imminent, he wants to be attended by a member of the clergy and given last rites. The fact that a particular individual chooses to be so treated does not justify that others be also so treated—whether they like it or not.

Is it possible to reconcile the conflicting fears and desires of the psychiatric protectionists and the psychiatric voluntarists? It is not only possible, it is easy: The solution for our dilemma lies ready-made in the Last Will—a legal mechanism people developed long ago for coping with an anticipated situation in which one's capacity to act is absent. Moreover, the model of the Last Will has already inspired the formation of an analogous instrument—namely, the Living Will. These two legal instruments help us to plan for death and incapacitating terminal illness. I propose that we create a third type of will: the Psychiatric Will.

However, before proceeding, I want to note that, at the present time, neither last wills nor living wills are protected against psychiatric nullification—that is, by having the maker of the will declared mentally incompetent at the time he executed the will. Many years ago, I described a mechanism for protecting a person's Last Will against posthumous psychiatric nullification by means of a mechanism similar to that suggested in this essay.[14] In short, the policy I propose offers protection from unwanted psychiatric meddling for both bodily and mentally ill persons on whom others may, in the future, want to impose unwanted treatments of some kind.

Many people want to be able to determine what will happen to their property after they die. The Last Will—or so-called Last Testament, the use of which is an ancient practice—enables us to do so, by extending our powers of control to a future situation in which we would no longer have any control. The Living Will meets a similar, though historically much more recent, contingency—namely, the desire to control the management of a lingering, painful, and absurdly expensive terminal illness, at a time when one may no longer be physically or mentally able to do so.[15] Executed while the individual is not disabled by illness, anticipating a future time when he might be, the Living Will directs those responsible for caring for its author to provide (extraordinary) life-sustaining measures for him, or to insure that such measures are withheld from him. To make such a legal instrument work, it is necessary, of course, that its implementation be backed by popular opinion and legal philosophy. The Last Will, as I noted, has received such backing since ancient times. In the United States, the Living Will receives such support now. The classic case is *Natanson v. Kline*, in which a Kansas court held that, "Anglo-American law starts with the premise of thorough-going self-determination. It follows that each man is considered to be the master of his own body, and he may, *if he be of sound mind*, expressly prohibit the performance of life-saving surgery."[16] In the same vein, an authoritative law review article, on "Compulsory Lifesaving Treatment for the Competent Adult," concludes:

> Every competent adult is free to reject life-saving medical treatment. This freedom is
> grounded, depending upon the patient's claim, either on the right to determine what

shall be done with one's body or the right of free religious exercise—both fundamental rights in the American scheme of personal liberty.[17]

The Psychiatric Will I propose rests on the same principle and seeks to extend it to psychiatric treatment. It asserts, in effect, that a competent American adult has (should have) a legally recognized right to reject involuntary psychiatric interventions that he may be deemed to require in the future, when, because of insanity, he may be declared/diagnosed to be incompetent to make decisions concerning his own welfare. I model the Psychiatric Will after the Living Will and, specifically, on the right of a Jehovah's Witness to reject life-saving blood transfusion as a medical treatment.[18]

Concerning the constitutionality of allowing Jehovah's Witnesses to reject blood transfusion, even when it may be lifesaving, the classic opinion is that written by Chief Justice (then Circuit Judge) Warren Burger in 1964. To buttress his conclusion, Burger recalled Justice Louis Brandeis' famous admonition:

> The makers of our Constitution sought to protect Americans in their beliefs, their thoughts, their emotions, and their sensations. They conferred, as against the Government, the right to be let alone—the most comprehensive of rights, and the right most valued by civilized man.[19]

To this oft-cited opinion, Burger added these—for our present purposes, decisive—words:

> Nothing in this utterance suggests that Justice Brandeis thought an individual possessed these rights only as to *sensible* beliefs, *valid* thoughts, *reasonable* emotions, or *well-founded* sensations. I suggest he intended to include a great many foolish, unreasonable, and even absurd ideas which do not conform, such as refusing medical treatment even at great risk.[20]

Because the First Amendment bars the government equally from imposing special burdens on, or extending special privileges to, members of one or another religious group, it follows that if Jehovah's Witnesses possess such far-reaching rights to reject what they consider to be unwanted medical interventions, so do we all.

Actually, the Jehovah's Witnesses' attitude toward blood transfusion constitutes a special case in a much larger class of instances in which individuals want to reject medical treatment, even when such treatment may be lifesaving (or life-prolonging, a distinction that may be difficult or impossible to make). The most obvious situation that comes to mind in this connection is that of the aged or incurably ill person who does not want his life prolonged by means of extraordinarily complex, invasive, or expensive medical interventions.[21] Already, several groups lobby on behalf of such persons to secure them a legally recognized "right to die." One such group, the "Society for the Right to Die," has drafted a model Living Will. I shall cite some portions of this Living Will, to illustrate its thrust and to indicate the form that a Psychiatric Will might take:

> Declaration made this_____ day of _____ month/year. I,_____
> _____, being of sound mind, willfully and voluntarily make known my
> desire that my dying shall not be artificially prolonged under the circumstances set
> forth below, do hereby declare: If at any time I should have an incurable injury,
> disease. . . . I direct that such [life sustaining] procedures be withheld or withdrawn
> and that I be permitted to die naturally. . . . In the absence of my ability to give
> directions regarding the use of such life-sustaining procedures, it is my intention that
> this declaration shall be honored by my family and physician(s) as the final expression
> of my legal right to refuse medical or surgical treatment.[22]

As I noted, where the person is conscious and rational, the courts have tended to accept the principle that an individual has a right to refuse medical treatment, even if the result is death. "*Even in an emergency situation,*" a medical ethicist emphasizes, "where death would ensue if treatment were not administered, the court . . . upheld a patient's refusal of treatment."[23] Since involuntary psychiatric interventions are rarely lifesaving—and, even if they were, in conformity with the foregoing ethical-legal principles, that would not be enough to justify their forcible imposition on unwilling clients—the *parens patriae* rationale for psychiatric coercions is gravely undermined by the evidence I have adduced. In fact, inasmuch as the Psychiatric Will bestows the right to reject psychiatric treatment on persons deemed—even by courts and psychiatrists—to be mentally competent and rational at the time of their making their decision against involuntary psychiatric interventions, it is difficult to see on what constitutional, moral, or political grounds Americans could be denied this right.

Let us keep in mind, also, that an impasse between the protagonists of two positions, each basing his policies on different premises, is not unique to the conflict about involuntary psychiatric interventions. The dilemma epitomized by the attitude of the Jehovah's Witness toward blood transfusion is helpful in this connection. In American law, this conflict has been resolved by adopting the policy that no adult should receive a blood transfusion against his will, and no one who wants to receive blood should be denied the benefits of this treatment (assuming that he has access to medical care and physicians deem the procedure necessary). It seems astonishing that a similar tactic of conflict resolution has not heretofore been proposed for dealing with the clash between the proponents and opponents of coercive psychiatry. I shall restate the conflict about commitment, so that the differing premises of the two protagonists are clearly articulated.

Many people—including virtually all psychiatrists and other mental health experts—fear the danger of a psychotic illness. These persons believe that mental illnesses exists, are "like any other illness," are amenable to modern psychiatric treatments, and that the effectiveness and legitimacy of the treatments are independent of the patient's consent to being treated. Accordingly, such persons seek protection from life-threatening mental illness and support the use of involuntary psychiatric interventions.

On the other hand, some people—including a few psychiatrists and other mental health experts—fear the literal danger of psychiatry more than the metaphoric danger of psychosis. Some of these persons also believe that mental illnesses do not exist and that psychiatric coercions are not treatments but tortures. Accordingly, such persons seek protection from the powers of psychiatry and advocate the abolition of involuntary psychiatric interventions.

Let me now apply the principles underlying the Last Will and the Living Will to the psychiatric contingency some people might want to anticipate and control. The imagery of acute psychosis, sketched earlier, represents the dreaded situation that some persons may want to anticipate and plan for. Since involuntary psychiatric confinement is a tradition-honored custom in modern societies, the situation such persons need to anticipate must be their own sudden madness, managed by others by means of commitment and coerced treatment. To forestall such an event, we need a mechanism enabling anyone reaching the age of maturity, who so desires, to execute a Psychiatric Will prohibiting his confinement in a mental hospital and his involuntary treatment for mental illness. Those failing to execute such a document before an actual encounter with coercive psychiatry would, of course, have the opportunity to do so as soon as they have regained their competence.

Because commitment entails the loss of liberty, the foregoing mechanism for its protection is weak, as it requires the affirmative assertion of a desire to do without involuntary psychiatric care. In the absence of such a declaration, the person would remain a potentially defenseless subject for psychiatric coercion. Although the adoption of such a policy would be a vast improvement over the present situation, a more powerful Psychiatric Will could be easily fashioned by inverting the right to be asserted in it. In the stronger version of the Psychiatric Will, a person would have to assert his desire to be the beneficiary of psychiatric coercion, should the need for it arise. This would leave everyone who has not executed a Psychiatric Will free from psychiatric coercion, much as we are free, without having to go to such troubles, of theological coercion.

Although the stronger version of the Psychiatric Will is theoretically more attractive, the long tradition of coercive paternalism may make the weaker version more immediately practical. In any case, no one who executes a Psychiatric Will would have to embrace or reject psychiatric interventions in their totality. On the contrary, some persons might wish to permit coerced hospitalization, but prohibit treatment by drugs or electroshock; others might wish to permit coerced drug therapy, but prohibit involuntary hospitalization. Only through a mechanism such as the Psychiatric Will could the responsibilities as well as the rights of the so-called seriously mentally ill be expanded.

In short, the adoption of the Psychiatric Will might put an end to the dispute about involuntary psychiatric interventions. Earnestly applied, such a policy should satisfy the demands of both the psychiatric protectionist and the psychiatric voluntarist. Surely, the psychiatric protectionist could not, in good faith, object to being frustrated in his therapeutic efforts by a person mentally competent to make binding decisions about his future—in this case, to prohibit personally unauthorized psychiatric assistance. Similarly, the psychiatric abolitionist could not, in good faith, object to being frustrated in his libertarian efforts by a person mentally competent to make binding decisions about his future—in this case, to authorize his own temporary (or not-so-temporary) psychiatric tutelage.

Moreover, the growing power of the Therapeutic State throughout the world suggests that the need for protecting the individual from medical-psychiatric intrusion will increase in the years ahead.[24] A Spanish law of 1980 is a straw in the wind that promises to blow down entire forests:

A new Spanish law has decreed that the bodies of deceased Spanish citizens belong to the state. Under this law the bodies may be used immediately upon death by hospitals for transplants without consultation with relatives. The only exemptions will be those who carried a card stating that they did not wish their bodies to be used in such a way.[25]

The mind of the insane has, of course, belonged to the state for a very long time already. And the statisticians of the Therapeutic State tell us that the proportion of such minds in the population is growing at an astounding rate.

It would be impossible to anticipate and articulate, in this essay, all of the consequences that might result from adopting the use of a Psychiatric Will. Still, some of its consequences are predictable.

Although my main goal in proposing a Psychiatric Will is to protect potential mental patients from unwanted psychiatric interventions, the Will would also protect therapists from some of the risks they now face in their relations with (involuntary) mental patients. This dual function of the Psychiatric Will is inherent in the fact that it is an instrument for transforming a status relationship into a contractual relationship.[26] Today, the psychiatrist faced with the task of caring for a seriously ill mental patient often finds himself in a Catch-22 type of situation: He is at risk for being sued both for confining and for failing to confine the patient, for using coercive treatment as well as for failing to use it. The Psychiatric Will, prospectively requesting or refusing involuntary psychiatric inter- ventions, would constitute a contract between the potential psychiatric patient and his potential psychiatrists: It would protect the former from psychiatric coercion or psychiatric neglect, and the latter from charges of unauthorized treatment or unprofessional neglect.

Lest these remarks appear too abstract, I offer herewith a typical scenario, illustrating the sort of risks against which the Psychiatric Will would protect psychiatrists.

A middle-aged, Roman Catholic, married executive, with three children all under ten years old, becomes disenchanted with his wife, falls in love with his twenty-year-old secretary, has an affair with her, and contemplates divorce. Overcome with conflict over the existential complexities in which he has become enmeshed, he becomes depressed, confesses all to his wife, and drops hints to her that perhaps it would be best for everyone if he killed himself. She persuades him to see a psychiatrist. The psychiatrist diagnoses our hypothetical patient to be suffering from a depression, prescribes antidepressant medication, and asks the patient to return for another appointment a week later. Reluctantly, the patient returns. The psychiatrist concludes that the patient's depression has worsened, recommends immediate psychiatric hospitalization, and informs both the patient and his wife that the danger of suicide is an important reason for this recommendation. The patient requests permission to go to his office to take care of some important business matters before checking into the hospital. He leaves, goes to his office, and shoots himself in the head. The wound is not fatal, but causes extensive brain damage that renders the patient a complete invalid. Should the patient's wife sue for malpractice, charging the psychiatrist with negligence for letting her husband leave the psychiatrist's office, she has a good chance of winning a large award. On the other hand, should the psychiatrist promptly commit the patient, the patient might quickly gain his release from the hospital and then sue the psychiatrist for false imprisonment and the damages he has suffered as a result of it. This litigation may also easily go against the psychiatrist. Were such an encounter to occur under the umbrella of a Psychiatric Will, the patient's prior acceptance or rejection of psychiatric coercion under such circumstances would protect the psychiatrist against the risk of employing or eschewing (as the case may be) involuntary psychiatric interventions.

As a practical matter, the availability of a Psychiatric Will would have no effect on those who choose, actively or passively, to accept involuntary psychiatric interventions. The consequences for those who choose to reject such interventions would depend on specific circumstances.

One large group of individuals who would be treated differently than they are at present is comprised of persons charged with serious crimes. Today, such persons are routinely subjected to pretrial psychiatric examinations to determine their competence to stand trial. Armed with a prohibitive Psychiatric Will, this tactic could be used only with the permission of the accused. The principle that a defendant is presumed to be competent to stand trial, like the principle that he is presumed to be innocent, would thus begin to be restored to the American criminal law. *Mutatis mutandis*, persons who commit crimes would have to be tried, and if guilty, punished, instead of being diverted into the psychiatric system.

Finally, individuals innocent of lawbreaking but deemed to be in need of psychiatric care would have to be persuaded that receiving such care would serve their best interests. If they refuse, they would, in Justice Louis Brandeis' words, have to be granted their "right to be let alone." Persons we deem in need of psychiatric help as well as those who claim that they want to help them would thus both be deprived of the option of coercing one another: The resulting tensions would generate a powerful impetus for developing fresh, non-coercive ways of dealing with the human predicaments we now mislabel as mental illnesses, and mismanage as psychiatric treatments.

11

Ex Parte Psychiatry

No man is free in doing evil. To prevent him is to set him free.

—Jacobin maxim

It is now widely accepted, especially by Americans, that confining lawbreakers in mental hospitals as insane, rather than in prisons as criminals, is a modern, scientific, Western practice. Nothing could be further from the truth. The practice is neither modern, nor scientific, nor typically Western; in fact, it more closely resembles the Oriental-despotic rejection of deviants than the Occidental-legal respect toward defendants. The following is a typical example.

In the years before the first World War, Grigorii Rasputin—whom history knows as the "mad monk," though he was neither mad nor a monk—was, after Nicholas and Alexandra, the most powerful person in Russia. As the Empress's most trusted friend and "therapist," he exercised enormous influence over her; and she, in turn, had virtually complete control over the weak and ineffectual Czar. Not surprisingly, Rasputin was widely hated and feared, and was eventually assassinated in 1916. However, there was a previous, failed attempt to kill him: In 1914, a woman named Chionya Gusyeva, dressed as a beggar, approached Rasputin in his home town of Pokrovskoe and, when Rasputin reached for his money, stabbed him in the lower abdomen. Rasputin survived. As for Gusyeva, she was treated exactly like countless Americans accused of crimes have been and continue to be treated:

> Gusyeva was arrested. . . . She announced that she had tried to kill Rasputin for abusing his so-called sainthood, for his heresies, and for raping a nun. The authorities felt it would be a mistake to put her on trial. After a short imprisonment she was conveniently declared insane and put in an asylum in Tomsk. Her relatives made repeated attempts to get her out, on the grounds that she had "got better," but the doctor in

173

charge insisted that she continued to display symptoms of "psychological disturbance and exalted religiosity." She did not get out until after the February Revolution.[1]

This procedure has all the earmarks of traditional Oriental despotism: It is arbitrary; it is unilateral, the defendant's "betters" deciding how best to deal with him; it is devoid of any mechanism for appealing the punishment; and, while defined as compassionate and humane (even medical and therapeutic), the charade simply serves the convenience of the defendant's adversaries.[2] Long ago, this paternalistic procedure for dealing with persons who disrupt the social order was grafted onto the tree of the American legal system: By pushing unwanted persons out on this limb, we ensure that they fall to their psychiatric deaths, while we bask in the glory of our therapeutic rationalizations.[3]

I regard the setting aside of a criminal trial and its replacement with psychiatric methods of punishing persons accused of crimes as one of psychiatry's most characteristic and most important social practices. Why? Because I value individual liberty and believe that a fair trial, conducted in public, is one of our most powerful safeguards against political tyranny, regardless of the tyrant's motives—to enslave and exploit his victim, or to protect and treat him.

There are, of course, many methods for determining guilt and punishing lawbreaking other than the criminal trial as practiced in contemporary English and American courts. Indeed, figuratively speaking, the phenomenon of obeying-disobeying rules may be said to begin at the organismic level, where it consists of following or transgressing biological rules: To survive as an *organism*, man must eat and drink what is nutritious or at least safe, and avoid eating and drinking what is nonnutritious or poisonous. On a higher, interpersonal level, we obey or disobey social rules: To survive as a *person*, man must observe certain rules or be punished for not doing so. The crucial difference between these two phenomena is that the deleterious consequences of violating biological rules are automatic—that is, do not require the intervention of human agents; whereas the deleterious consequences of violating social rules are not automatic, but require the intervention of human agents. Furthermore, because the crux of social life is obeying and disobeying rules, all of us, at all times, are both potential rule-followers and potential rule-breakers. As modern sociologists have noted, in an important sense, the violations of rules and their punishments *define* what the rules really are. This raises two simple but all-important questions: How do we know or ascertain that a rule has been broken? And, having ascertained it, by whom and by what means is the rule breaker punished? A brief glance at history gives us the answers we need for our present purposes.

In the Judeo-Christian worldview, history begins with a crime and a punishment: The crime is Adam's and Eve's disobedience of God (the Fall); and the punishment is expulsion from the Garden (a finite life or death). My point here is not to rehearse this familiar legend but to note that these legendary criminals never received a trial, much less a fair one. Nor was there, in the context in which the crime was set, any need for a trial. God, the Perfect Autocrat, knew when man was good and when he was bad. He needed no one else and nothing else to mete out justice: His judgment and punishment were by definition just. When absolute monarchs—emperors, kings, czars—ruled by divine decree, they decided, in a similarly autocratic-despotic manner, who was to be punished and how, and the punishment was, by definition, just.

But unlike gods, human beings are not omniscient. Thus, long ago it must have occurred to people that a person might be accused falsely and punished unjustly. To determine whether an alleged rule-violation has, in fact, occurred, more than accusation is needed; the accusation must be true. To punish justly, more than superior power is needed; the punishment must be fair and fitting. Out of such sentiments arose various mechanisms for adjudicating offenses, among them our Anglo-American concept of due process, and the adversarial method of ascertaining truth in courts of law on which it is rests.

In one form or another, trial is an ancient and virtually universal institution. In this connection, let us remember that Socrates and Jesus, Servetus and Galileo, witches and heretics, were tried. To be sure, by our standards, these trials were not fair. But they were, morally and politically, better than no trial at all—better than people being massacred in the middle of the night by a despot's deputies; better than people disappearing, without a trace, into concentration camps or the Gulag; better than people being dispatched, in a mockery of due process, to prisons called mental hospitals.

To appreciate what, from a moral and libertarian point of view, is bad about despotic law enforcement, whether of the Oriental or psychiatric kind, we must be clear about what is good about the Anglo-American idea of a fair trial. As I see it, the crux of what is bad about the former is that it is *non-adversarial*, and the crux of what is good about the latter is that it is *adversarial*. As I emphasized, when God punishes the biblical Israelites, He weighs the evidence, He decides, He metes out the penalty—and that's that. This model of administering justice—which we may call religious, despotic, paternalistic, or therapeutic—has prevailed in most societies through most of history. Pitted against it—frequently assailed, but always beloved by all who treasure personal liberty and responsibility—stands the adversarial model. Although not as old as the despotic method, the adversarial procedure is also of ancient origin.

However, the history of criminal trials as systems of social control does not concern us here. What does concern us is that the modern Anglo-American concept of a fair trial consists of three basic parts: prosecution, defense, and judge/jury. In effect, the trial is a contest between prosecuting attorney and defense attorney: They engage in a protracted argument or debate whose outcome they themselves cannot decide. The outcome of the contest is decided by judge and jury who, for their part, cannot join the debate; instead, their task is to conduct the proceedings and decide the outcome according to certain strict rules.

To be sure, we could decide that we do not like this system of adjudicating criminal responsibility; that we no longer believe that some persons charged with crimes are guilty and others innocent; and that those not proved guilty are entitled to remain free and unmolested by the government. But we cannot, it seems to me, continue to regard more and more lawbreakers as legally innocent, morally guilty, and fit for indefinite psychiatric imprisonment—and hope to preserve our hard-won political liberties.

In the East, where the right to property was never a fundamental value, the right to personal liberty never developed. In the West, where the two rights developed in tandem, both rights remain fragile and endangered— by collectivist-statist political subversion and by psychiatric-therapeutic erosion. This psychiatric erosion began in England in the eighteenth century, gathered momentum during the nineteenth, and, it seems to me, reached a critical level in the United States in the years following the Second World War. Today, in our typical psychiatrized nontrial, the prosecution does not prosecute, the defense does not defend, and the judge does not preside over a trial; instead, all three parties join in pretending to protect the defendant while, in fact, they are destroying him. The result is a regression to an ancient, religious-despotic criminal procedure where the guilt of the defendant was assumed from the outset and the "trial" was merely the ceremonial purging of evil from the community. This turning away from the heavy existential demands of the adversarial criminal trial is evident already in many nineteenth-century insanity trials, including the classic so-called trial of Daniel McNaughton. I say "so-called" because, as I intend to show, McNaughton was never *really* tried: his trial was a charade, a mere formality.

The facts of the case are briefly as follows. On 20 January 1843, Daniel McNaughton shot and killed Edward Drummond, Sir Robert Peel's private secretary. Believing himself victimized by the Tories, McNaughton wanted to shoot Peel, but mistook Drummond for the home secretary. For reasons that need not concern us here—but principally because of the mounting aversion against the death penalty in Victorian England—counsels for both defense and prosecution, as well as the judges, agreed that McNaughton was insane and should be found not guilty by reason of insanity.[4]

The proceedings against McNaughton began on 2 February 1843, when the Lord Chief Justice of England, Lord Abinger, asked him to plead: "How say you, prisoner, are you guilty or not guilty?" After a pause, McNaughton answered: "I am guilty of firing." Lord Abinger then asked: "By that, do you mean to say you are not guilty of the remainder of the charge; that is, of intending to murder Mr. Drummond?" "Yes," replied McNaughton.[5]

Revealingly, Lord Abinger did not ask McNaughton whether he intended to murder Sir Robert Peel. Instead, a plea of "not guilty" was entered on his behalf. A long trial ensued at which much lay testimony was given in support of the view that McNaughton knew perfectly well what he was doing, that he intended to kill Peel, but merely shot the wrong man. For example, Benjamin Weston, an "office porter" who happened to be on the scene, testified that "the prisoner drew the pistol very deliberately, but at the same time very quickly. As far as I can judge, it was a very cool, deliberate act."[6] Others, among them a surgeon named James Douglas, testified similarly:

I am a surgeon, residing at Glasgow. I am in the habit of giving lectures on anatomy. I recognize the prisoner as having been a student of mine last summer. I had the opportunities of speaking to him almost every day; I merely spoke to him on the subject of anatomy. He seemed to understand it. . . . I never observed anything to lead me to suppose his mind was disordered.[7]

Nine "medical gentlemen"—led by Dr. E. T. Monro, one of the most prominent alienists of the day—then testified,

> all emphasizing that his [McNaughton's] delusions of persecution meant that "his moral liberty was destroyed." The Crown presented no medical evidence to rebut this, even though McNaughton had obtained firearms, had watched his victim for several days, and had waited till his victim's back was turned.[8]

At the conclusion of the testimony, the chief prosecutor addressed the jury and asked it to find the defendant not guilty by reason of insanity:

> SOLICITOR GENERAL: Gentlemen of the jury, after the intimation I have received from the Bench I feel that I should not be properly discharging my duties to the Crown and to the public if I asked you to give your verdict in this case *against* the prisoner. . . . This unfortunate man, at the time he committed the act was labouring under insanity; and, of course, if he were so, he would be entitled to his acquittal.[9]

I emphasize the word *against* to indicate that the prosecutor considered the decision to execute McNaughton as being against him, and the decision to imprison him for life as being *not against* him. But McNaughton never asked for this. Clearly, it was the lawyers and judges, not McNaughton, who were disturbed by the prospect of his being put to death. And so, in the end, the chief judge, C. J. Tindal, instructed the jury to bring in a verdict of not guilty by reason of insanity, leading to this colloquy:

> C. J. TINDAL: . . . If you think you ought to hear the evidence more fully, in that case I will state it to you, and leave the case in your hands. Probably, however, sufficient has now been laid before you, and you will say whether you want further information.
> FOREMAN OF THE JURY: We require no more, my Lord.
> C. J. TINDAL: If you find the prisoner not guilty, say on the ground of insanity, in which case proper care will be taken of him.
> FOREMAN: We find the prisoner not guilty, on the grounds of insanity.[10]

It is a shameful travesty of justice that, ever since 1843, historians and scholars, psychiatrists and lawyers, have spoken and written about the "McNaughton trial," inasmuch as there never was a McNaughton *trial*. Calling what happened in court to McNaughton a criminal trial—formally designating it as "The Queen Against Daniel McNaughton"—is an Orwellian untruth: The Queen did not proceed *against* McNaughton, she proceeded *for* him, so that, as the judge himself phrased it, "proper care will be taken of him." With that phrase, Judge Tindal made it clear to the jury that, as modern American slang would have it, McNaughton will be given the treatment.

However, there are many circumstances quite unlike McNaughton's, where a person is genuinely disabled and vulnerable, and where the courts take an honest, nonhypocritical cognizance of that fact. Thus, both English and American law recognizes certain circumstances where judicial authorities do not seek to prosecute and punish a person, but endeavor rather to protect him—from his own disability and from those who might take advantage of his vulnerability. Called an *ex parte* proceeding, the procedure is defined as "a judicial proceeding . . . taken or granted at the instance and for *the benefit of one party only, and without notice to, or contestation by, any person adversely interested.*"[11]

This is precisely how the McNaughton trial was handled. The judicial authorities did not solicit McNaughton's consent for treating him as a helpless infant-person, who could not care for himself and hence could not be prosecuted for a crime. Instead, all of the *dramatis personae*—that is, prosecutor, defense counsel, judges, and jury—relinquished their customary judicial roles and assumed instead the duties of guardians. Thus, the legal proceeding responsible for McNaughton's fate after he shot Drummond should have been called *Ex parte the Queen, in the matter of the mad Daniel McNaughton.* Ironically, like Daniel McNaughton, Queen Victoria was a party to this proceeding in name only. Actually, she was angry with the conduct of the trial, maintaining that it is absurd to suggest that a British subject who deliberately sets out to assassinate one of her ministers is not guilty of a crime. Her displeasure with the (non)trial generated the historic hearing before the House of Lords that led to the adoption of what we now call "the McNaughton rule."

Did McNaughton's self-appointed guardians help their ward? If saving McNaughton from the gallows is considered help, then the answer is yes. If we believe there are fates worse than death—especially when that is what the subject wants for himself —then the answer is no. In any case, *de jure*, McNaughton was treated as if he had been insane when he shot Drummond. *De facto*, he was treated as if he had been, was, and will always remain insane. McNaughton was confined as a madman for the remaining twenty-one years of his life. He died in Broadmoor (the first so-called hospital for the criminally insane in England) in 1864.

I should note here that by the time McNaughton came to trial, this method of disposing of capital cases was not unusual in England. In his study of Victorian insanity trials, Roger Smith comments: "In practice, a warrant of removal to a criminal asylum usually meant a permanent removal. It was extremely difficult to attribute 'recovery' to someone who had shown potential for violence."[12] That is an understatement. It was plain as day that the real purpose of the insanity verdict was imprisonment for life in an insane asylum without the possibility of parole, and that such a fate was a terrible punishment indeed. For example, Dr. Forbes Winslow, a leading Victorian alienist, cited the terrors of the insanity verdict to tout the advantages of the insanity defense:

> To talk of a person escaping the extreme penalty of the law on the plea of Insanity, as one being subjected to no kind or degree of *punishment*, is a perfect mockery of truth and perversion of language. Suffer no punishment! He is exposed to the severest pain and torture of body and mind that can be inflicted upon a human creature short of being publicly strangled upon the gallows. If the fact be doubted, let a visit be paid to that dreadful *den* at Bethlehem Hospital . . . where the criminal portion of the establishment are confined like wild beasts in an iron cage![13]

Thus, almost 150 years ago (in 1858), psychiatrists hit upon this clever double-talk for advertising the asylum: For the non-criminal, the insane asylum is a *hospital*, the ideal place for treating mental illness; for the criminal, it is a *prison*, the ideal place for storing "wild beasts."

Surveying the fate of insanity acquittees serving life sentences in insane asylums, Smith wryly observes that "medical superintendents accepted their custodial role."[14] Again that is putting the matter mildly. Actually, Victorian "medical men" vied for the privilege of being the executioners of such brutal punishments. Today, the executioners are called "forensic psychiatrists," and they vie for that privilege even more intensely.

The reader must keep in mind, in this connection, that the criminals saved by psychiatry in the nineteenth century stayed incarcerated until they died, often for many decades. John W. Hinckley, Jr., currently the most famous American insanity acquittee, has already spent more than ten years behind therapeutic bars, and his cure is nowhere in sight. Compare this with what happens to convicted murderers in the United States: "Those released from prison [in the 1980s] for murder and nonnegligent manslaughter served a median of 78 months in confinement."[15] With capital punishment virtually abolished, and prison-time served for murder shorter than ever, "psychiatric justice" is even more punitive and more unjust today than it was a century ago.

The particular psychiatric practice I have considered in this essay— namely, the pretrial psychiatric examination of defendants, the legal-medical judgment that they are mentally unfit to stand trial, and their subsequent psychiatric incarceration—hinges on, and is an integral part of, the psychiatrist's power to hospitalize persons against their will. Psychiatrists have always had, and continue to have, a veritable love affair with the practice of coercion—which they equate with, and peddle as, compassion; reciprocally, legislators, lawyers, and lay persons have had a love affair with submission to psychiatric coercion—which they equate with, and peddle as, care. So long as this collusion continues—so long as most people believe that psychiatrists are entitled to exercise power over persons labeled "mental patients"—psychiatrists will gladly exercise such power, and people will gullibly submit to it. Hence, it is naive as well as foolish, though no doubt self-satisfying, for politicians, physicians, and the press to indulge in periodic outbursts of indignation at psychiatric "abuses."[16]

It is the very legitimacy of the psychiatrist's power—his moral and legal right to intimidate, much less to imprison—that requires our scrutiny. And, in my opinion, our condemnation and rejection.

Epilogue

Healthy people are sick people who don't know it. . . . "Health" is a word which we could just as well erase from our vocabularies. For me there are only people more or less sick of more or less numerous diseases progressing at a more or less rapid rate.

—Jules Romains, *Knock*

Priests used to be in the habit of making pronouncements about demons and angels, the bad climate in hell, and the beautiful music in heaven. How did people view such religious claims in the past? How do we view them today? As God-given truths or bombastic slang?

For two hundred years, psychiatrists have been in the habit of making similarly preposterous pronouncements about the epidemiology of mental illnesses and their therapeutic powers to prevent and cure them. Claiming that everyone is mentally ill came as easily to the lips of the most respected psychiatrists as claiming that all sinners go to hell came to the lips of the most revered clergymen. How do we view such psychiatric claims? As scientific truths or bombastic slang?

For a tiny corps of critics—psychiatric atheists, as it were—the scientific pretensions of mad doctors are self-evidently phony, on par with the pretensions of mesmerists and phrenologists. For the general public as well as the pillars of society—including the leaders in science, medicine, law, and politics —the discoveries, diagnoses, treatments, and theories of psychiatry are just as valid as those of any other branch of human knowledge. One of the main reasons for this is the hypnotic effect of psychiatric slang, lulling people into the false belief that if something is called a disease it is a disease, and if it is called a treatment it is a treatment. When even a linguist of Richard A. Spears' sophistication and standing—he is professor of linguistics at Northwestern University and the editor of several major anthologies on slang—softens and thus undoes his recognition of psychiatry as a culturally validated semantic charade, we are confronted with the full force, irresistible in its time and place, of conventional wisdom.

"A culture's vocabulary," states Spears, "contains a record of the culture's values, fears, hostilities, and mistakes."[1] Note that Spears brackets slang terms and technical terms as serving a similar purpose:

"Many slang terms, euphemisms, colloquial terms, and technical terms came into use so that people could avoid writing or saying prohibited terms for unpleasant subjects."[2] Apropos of what he calls "avoidance terms," exemplified by locutions intended to avoid saying the name of God, Spears writes:

> Another such class includes the classical medical avoidances found in the "phobia" and "mania" terms. *Most* of the disabilities contained in this nomenclature are easily describable in ordinary English, and *very few of them* constitute specific disorders with well-defined *symptoms* or *treatment*.[3]

Spears's qualification in the passage above is like saying that *very few* of the theological statements about the climatic conditions in hell are meteorologically sound. But *none* is. And the same goes for *all* of the mental illnesses manufactured by means of Greco-Latin roots, prefixes, and suffixes (the "manias," "philias," and "phobias"). By conceding that some phobias are genuine illnesses, Spears leaves the door ajar enough for the conquering armies of medicalization to march right through it. Either we say that no phobia is a disease, because being afraid of something is simply not the sort of thing that can be constitutive of a bodily disease, or we let certain authorities decide which phobias are, and which are not, diseases. Agoraphobia, gamophobia, homophobia, opiophobia, syphilophobia, zoophobia—which is, and which is not, a disease?

To be sure, fear and avoidance may be a part and parcel of having a disease. Any reasonable person suffering from osteoporosis would be afraid of falling, and hence avoid ice skating as a hobby. Similarly, any reasonable person dining in a restaurant in Mexico would be afraid of acquiring an intestinal infection, and hence avoid drinking tap water. Calling a fear exaggerated, unfounded, irrational, or morbid does not remove "it" from the class of phenomena we call "fears"; but fears, unlike bodily lesions, are not the building blocks of diseases. Nevertheless, Spears leaves open the possibility that the psychiatric nomenclature is, medically speaking, not a complete hoax. But it is. Which is not to say that the phenomena to which psychiatric terms refer are not real; they are real, indeed, just as real as the phenomena to which medical terms refer. Spear's own example is helpful here: "A young man might use the term 'goobers' among his peers, 'pimples' with his parents, 'acne' with his doctor, and 'acne vulgaris' in a Health Sciences term paper."[4]

Similarly, we have a wide range of words, phrases, and figures of speech from which to choose if we want to describe the fears and hatreds, the passions and perplexities, disappointments and despairs that are the lot of men, women, and children. We can choose to use ordinary words or psychiatric terms. Our choice points inexorably toward the ultimate question about language as our tool: What is it for? Different philosophers have offered different answers. Some said the purpose of language is to discover and declare truths. Others—Nietzsche in particular—maintained that its purpose is to lie. I suggest that its purpose is to do both, depending on what we want it to do.

We can use language to understand the world around us and communicate to others what we know and think. Or we can use it to obscure what is self-evident but embarrassing, deny what we know is true but painful, and conceal from others what we know and think. No one uses, or can use, language in only one of these ways. When we depend on the Other, we use language mainly to flatter him, and to justify and validate his beliefs and behavior. When we dominate the Other, we use language mainly to flatter ourselves, and to justify and validate our own beliefs and behavior.

Jefferson was right when he observed that "It is error alone which needs the support of government. Truth can stand by itself."[5] But where? Truth is veracity, not force. Against force, truth is powerless. Amidst people indifferent to truth, fearful of it, hostile to it, truth has no place. In short, truth can stand only where it will not be expelled as a trespasser—in the remote, politically neutral, regions of the hard sciences; in the intimate, but politically insignificant, retreats of the relations among equals; in the cracks and crevices of everyday life, where it poses no threat to normal social intercourse; and, most enduringly and most securely, in books and in libraries.

Notes

Introduction

1. S. Freud, "Psychical (or Mental) Treatment" [1905], in the *Standard Edition of the Complete Psychological Works of Sigmund Freud*, 24 vols. (London: Hogarth Press, 1953–74: 283 (hereafter cited as SE).
2. Editorial, "British psychiatry at 150," *The Lancet* 338 (28 September 1991):785.
3. M. Polanyi, "Life's Irreducible Structures" [1968], in, M. Polanyi *Knowing and Being: Essays by Michael Polanyi*, ed. Marjorie Grene (Chicago: University of Chicago Press, 1969), 238.
4. Ibid.
5. M. Freudenheim, "New Law to Bring Wider Job Rights for Mentally Ill," *New York Times*, 23 September 1991, pp. A1 & D4.
6. W. Rogers, "The Congressional Record" [1935], in *A Will Rogers Treasury: Reflections and Observations*, ed. B. B. Sterling and F. N. Sterling (New York: Bonanza Books, 1982), 256.
7. M. Freudenheim, "New Law," pp. A1 & D4.
8. M. Freudenheim, "At Work, a New Deal for the Mentally Ill," *Wall Street Journal*, 24 September 1991, p. A9.
9. M. J. Goldman, "Kleptomania: Making Sense Out of Nonsense," *American Journal of Psychiatry* 148 (August 1991): 986–96.
10. Ibid., 986 emphasis added.
11. See, generally, T. S. Szasz, *Insanity: The Idea and Its Consequences* (New York: Wiley, 1987).
12. C. Miller, "Course Offers Cure for Shoplifting," *Syracuse Herald-Journal*, 17 October 1991, p. B1.
13. Ibid., emphasis added.
14. L. Bien, "Addicted Shoppers Attempt to Buy Happiness," *Syracuse Herald-Journal*, 23 October 1991, p. C1.
15. Ibid., C3.
16. American Psychiatric Association, *Diagnostic and Statistical Manual of Mental Disorders of the American Psychiatric Association (DSM-III-R)*, 3rd ed. - rev. (Washington, D. C.: American Psychiatric Association, 1987), 255.
17. Ibid., 269.
18. Ibid., 283.
19. Ibid., 293.
20. Ibid., 316.
21. R. Karel, "Controversy Follows DWI Acquittal Based on Premenstrual Syndrome Defense," *Psychiatric News* 26 (6 September 1991): 16–18.
22. Ibid., 18.
23. Ibid.
24. See T. S. Szasz, *Insanity*, 9–98.
25. See, R. Pear, "Federal Auditors Report Rise in Abuses in Medical Billing," *New York Times*, 20 December 1991, pp. A1 & B6.
26. For a marvelous parody of the APA's *furor diagnosticus*, see D. A. Levy, "A Proposed Category for the *Diagnostic and Statistical Manual of Mental Disorders*

(DSM): Pervasive Labeling Disorder," *Journal of Humanistic Psychology* 32 (Winter 1992): 121–25.

27. T. S. Szasz, "Diagnoses Are Not Diseases," *The Lancet* 338 (December 1991): 1574–76.

Chapter 1. Shakespeare's Plays

1. W. Farnham, "Introduction," in W. Shakespeare, *The Tragedy of Hamlet, Prince of Denmark*, ed. W. Farnham (Baltimore: Penguin Books, 1957), 17.
2. Ibid.
3. All references are to the Penguin edition cited above and are to act, scene, and line.
4. W. Shakespeare, *A Midsummer Night's Dream*, ed. W. Farnham (Baltimore: Penguin Books, 1957), 5.1. 7–8.

Chapter 2. The Contemporary Scene

1. See, T. S. Szasz, *The Myth of Mental Illness: Foundations of a Theory of Personal Conduct* (1961; rev. ed., New York: Harper & Row, 1974), 32–38.
2. See, P. Craddock, "The Art and Craft of Faking: Copying, Embellishing, and Transforming," in, *Fake? The Art of Deception*, ed. M. Jones (Berkeley and Los Angeles: University of California Press, 1990).
3. See, T. S. Szasz, *Anti-Freud: Karl Kraus's Criticism of Psychiatry and Psychoanalysis* (1976; reprint, Syracuse: Syracuse University Press, 1990), and R. Monk, *Wittgenstein: The Duty of Genius* (New York: Penguin, 1991), 357.
4. S. Freud "Freud's Metapsychology Revisited," *Social Casework* 66 (March 1985):150.
5. Sir W. Scott, *Marmion: A Tale of Flodden Field*, in *Scott's Marmion*, ed. H. E. Coblentz (1808; reprint, New York: American Book Company, 1911), canto 6, stanza 17, p. 169.
6. J. Leff, "Schizophrenia in the Melting Pot," *Nature* 353 (24 October 1991): 693.
7. T. S. Szasz, *The Myth of Mental Illness* and *Insanity*.
8. J. Leff, "Schizophrenia," 694, emphasis added.
9. T.S. Szasz, "Diagnoses Are Not Diseases," 1574–76.
10. J.R. Smythies, "Wittgenstein's Paranoia," *Nature* 350 (7 March 1991): 9, emphasis added.
11. Ibid.
12. See, M. Eliade, ed., *The Encyclopedia of Religion* (New York: Macmillan, 1987), vol. 5, pp. 563–66.
13. Its scriptural source is 1 Cor. 13: 1, where St. Paul refers to "the tongues of men and angels." The Holy Bible, Revised Standard Version (New York: Meridian, 1962).
14. *Webster's Third New International Dictionary*, unabridged (Springfield, Mass.: G. & C. Merriam Co., 1961).
15. *New Catholic Encyclopedia* (Washington, D.C.: Catholic University of America, 1967), vol. 6, p. 473.
16. L. E. Hinsie and J. Shatzky, *Psychiatric Dictionary* (New York: Oxford University Press, 1953), 241.
17. J. M. Meth, "Exotic Psychiatric Syndromes," in *American Handbook of Psychiatry*, 2d ed., ed. S. Arieti and E. B. Brody (New York: Basic Books, 1974), 3:728.

18. H. I. Kaplan and B. J. Sadock, "Typical Signs and Symptoms of Psychiatric Illness," in H. I. Kaplan and B. J. Sadock, *Comprehensive Textbook of Psychiatry / V* (Baltimore: Williams & Wilkins, 1985), 1:472.

19. *The American Heritage Illustrated Encyclopedic Dictionary* (Boston: Houghton Mifflin, 1987), 716.

20. *The New Encyclopedia Britannica*, 15th ed. (Chicago: Encyclopedia Britannica, 1990), 11:842.

21. W. J. Samarin, *Tongues of Men and Angels: The Religious Language of Pentecostalism* (New York: Macmillan, 1972), xi.

22. 1 Cor. 1: 19–28.

23. W. J. Samarin, *Tongues of Men and Angels,* 13, 14.

24. Sir M. Roth, "Schizophrenia and the Theories of Thomas Szasz," *British Journal of Psychiatry* 129 (October 1976): 319.

25. T. S. Szasz, *Schizophrenia: The Sacred Symbol of Psychiatry* (1976; reprint, Syracuse: Syracuse University Press, 1988).

26. S. Rochester and J. R. Martin, *Crazy Talk: A Study of the Discourse of Schizophrenic Speakers* (New York: Plenum Press, 1979), 2–3.

27. Ibid., 7.

28. See, American Psychiatric Association, *Diagnostic and Statistical Manual of Mental Disorders of the American Psychiatric Association (DSM-III-R)*, 3rd ed., -rev., (Washington, D. C.: American Psychiatric Association, 1987), and T. J. Resnick and I. Lapin, "Language Disorders in Childhood," *Psychiatric Annals* 21 (December 1991): 709–16.

29. Resnick and Lapin, "Language Disorders," 716.

30. P. P. Wiener, ed., *Dictionary of the History of Ideas: Studies of Selected Pivotal Ideas,* 5 vols. (New York: Scribner's, 1973).

31. R. Williams, *Keywords: A Vocabulary of Culture and Society*, rev. ed. (New York: Oxford University Press, 1976).

32. H. L. Mencken, *The American Language: An Inquiry Into the Development of English in the United States,* 1 vol. abridged ed. (New York: A. A. Knopf, 1977), 702.

33. Our rich and revealing vocabulary of slang words for psychiatrists, which distinguishes them from real doctors, supports this thesis. Here are some examples: *bug doctor, head doctor, loco doctor, nut doctor, psycho, squirrel, strait man.*

34. American Psychiatric Association, DSM-III.

35. American Psychiatric Association, DSM-III-R.

36. N. Postman, *Crazy Talk, Stupid Talk* (New York: Delta, 1976), 57–58.

37. S. Freud, *The Psychopathology of Everyday Life* [1901], in SE 6.

38. Ibid., xiii–xiv.

39. I have argued this thesis in depth in several books, especially *The Myth of Mental Illness* and *Insanity.*

40. T. S. Szasz, *The Myth of Mental Illness,* 11–13.

Chapter 3. Dictionaries of Deviance

1. American Psychiatric Association, *DSM-III.*

2. American Psychiatric Association, *DSM-III-R,* xvii.

3. American Psychiatric Association, *DSM-IV Options Book: Work in Progress* (Washington, D. C.: American Psychiatric Association, 1991).

4. M. Zimmerman, "Is DSM-IV Needed At All?" Letters to the Editor, *Archives of General Psychiatry* 47 (October 1991): 974–76.
5. "Citing 'Retard' Slur, Group Changes Name," *New York Times*, 28 October 1991, p. A14.
6. I have omitted the Axes and Code Numbers.
7. See also Nicotine dependence.
8. Terms such as *alcohol abuse* and *drug abuse* are examples of the *language abuse* that infects our contemporary discourse about using drugs. We call the man who beats his wife a *wife abuser*: He harms another person. We call the man who smokes marijuana a *drug abuser*: But he does not harm marijuana. To the contrary, so-called drug abusers take good care not to abuse the drugs they consider precious. Although we *say* that such a person abuses drugs, we *mean* that he abuses himself. See generally, T. S. Szasz, *Our Right to Drugs: The Case for a Free Market* (New York: Praeger, 1992).
9. There are a vast number of slang and jargon terms for addiction to various drugs and for the persons who use such drugs, which I do not include in this list. See, R. A. Spear, *The Slang and Jargon of Drugs and Drink* (Metuchen, N.J.: Scarecrow Press, 1986).
10. Most of the "manias" and "phobias" are listed, respectively, under *mania* and *phobia*; those in common usage, like agoraphobia, are listed twice, alphabetically as well as under *phobia*.
11. The synonyms for malingering are from J. E. Schmidt, *Dictionary of Medical Slang and Related Esoteric Expressions* (Springfield, IL: Charles C. Thomas, 1959), 95.
12. As there is no object, idea, or behavior for which a person may not develop an excessive or irrational love or passion, there are a potentially infinite number of manias; and, mutatis mutandis, of phobias. The manias, philias, and phobias (in List 1) are edited, and slightly expanded, versions of those listed in *-Ologies & -Isms*, 3rd ed., by Laurence Urdang (Detroit: Gale Research, 1986).
13. Adapted from R. J. Campbell, *Psychiatric Dictionary*, 5th ed. (New York: Oxford University Press, 1981).
14. As there is no object, idea, or behavior of which a person may not be "abnormally" afraid, there are a potentially infinite number of phobias.
15. Adapted from R. J. Campbell, *Psychiatric Dictionary*.
16. H. L. Mencken, *The American Language: An Inquiry Into the Development of English in the United States*, 1 vol. abr. ed. (New York: Alfred A. Knopf, 1977), 353.
17. Ibid., 271.

Chapter 4. Dictionaries of Drunkenness

1. H. L. Mencken, *The American Language* 264.
2. Ibid., 268.
3. B. Franklin, "The Drinkers Dictionary," in *The Drinker's Dictionary & Other Useful Information on the Joys of Wine, Women, & Song* (Grosse Pointe, Mich.: Junto, A Private Press, 1965), 6–34.
4. See, C. Larson, "The Drinkers Dictionary," *American Speech* 12 (April 1937): 87–92; and, L. Pound, "Franklin's 'Drinkers Dictionary' Again," 15 (February 1940): 103–105.
5. J. Goodman, Jr, "Introduction," in, *The Drinker's Dictionary*, ix.

6. Larson, "The Drinkers Dictionary," 88.
7. B. Franklin, "Reflections on Drinking" (an undated letter), in, "The Drinkers Dictionary," 37–38.
8. Medical and scientific journals publish articles on the genetic causes of, or predispositions to, drunkenness (alcoholism) with the same certain knowledge that "it" is a disease as they publish articles on the genetic aspects of cystic fibrosis or diabetes. See, for example, C. Holden, "Probing the Complex Genetics of Alcoholism," *Science* 11 (January 1991): 163–64.
9. Larson, "The Drinkers Dictionary" 89.
10. Franklin, "The Drinkers Dictionary," 7–8.
11. See, Szasz, *Our Right to Drugs*, 31–58.
12. B. Franklin, "The Drinkers Dictionary."
13. E. Wilson, "The Lexicon of Prohibition," in *The American Earthquake: A Documentary of the Twenties and Thirties* (Garden City, N.Y.: Doubleday Anchor, 1958), 89–91.
14. Ibid., 91.
15. This dictionary is the product of my own compilation. I have incorporated in it many of the terms for drunkenness listed in the *Dictionary of American Slang*, 2nd supp. ed., ed. H. Wentworth and S. B. Flexner (New York: Thomas Y. Crowell, 1975), 634–35.

Chapter 5. The Religion Called "Psychiatry"

1. O. W. Holmes, quoted in, L. W. Levy, *Treason Against God: A History of the Offense of Blasphemy* (New York: Schocken, 1981), x.
2. T. Jefferson, "Thomas Jefferson to Thomas Jefferson Randolph," 24 November 1808, in *Jefferson's Letters*, arranged by W. Whitman, (Eau Claire, Wisc.: E. M. Hale, n.d.), 249.
3. T. S. Szasz, *The Myth of Psychotherapy: Mental Healing as Religion, Rhetoric, and Repression* (1978; reprinted, Syracuse: Syracuse University Press, 1988).
4. See, T. S. Szasz, *The Ethics of Psychoanalysis: The Theory and Method of Autonomous Psychotherapy* (1965; reprinted Syracuse: Syracuse University Press, 1988).
5. S. Freud, "Postscript to the Question of Lay Analysis" [1927], in SE 20; 252.
6. S. Freud, *Introductory Lectures on Psychoanalysis* [1916–1917], in SE 16; 389.
7. S. Freud, *New Introductory Lectures on Psychoanalysis* [1932], in SE 22; 152.
8. S. Freud, *The Complete Letters of Sigmund Freud to Wilhelm Fliess, 1887–1904*, trans. and ed. J. M. Masson. (Cambridge: Harvard University Press, 1985), 18–19; emphasis added.
9. See, T. S. Szasz, *Anti-Freud: Karl Kraus's Criticism of Psychoanalysis and Psychiatry* (1976; reprint Syracuse: Syracuse University Press, 1990).
10. K. Kraus, quoted in ibid., 103, 117.
11. Freud to Oskar Pfister, 9 February 1909, in E. Jones, *The Life and Work of Sigmund Freud*, 3 vols., (New York: Basic Books, 1953–1957), 2:440.
12. S. Freud, *The Future of an Illusion* [1927], in SE 21; 36.
13. S. Freud, *The Psychopathology of Everyday Life* [1901], in SE 6; 259; emphasis in original.
14. S. Freud, *The Future of an Illusion*, SE 21:36.
15. Ibid., 53, 56.

16. S. Freud, *Civilization and Its Discontents* [1929], in SE 21; 113, and *Introductory Lectures on Psychoanalysis* [1916-1917], in SE:16; 181.
17. S. Freud, quoted in, Jones, *The Life and Work of Sigmund Freud* 3; 359.

Chapter 6. Mental Illness and Mental Incompetence

1. *Zinermon v. Burch*, 494 U.S. 113 (1990), p. 118.
2. Ibid., 119.
3. Ibid., 121.
4. Ibid., 135, emphasis in original.
5. Ibid., 133.
6. B. J. Winick, "Voluntary Hospitalization after *Zinermon v. Burch*," *Psychiatric Annals* 21(October 1991: 584-89).
7. Ibid., 585.
8. R. S. Rock, M. A. Jacobson, and R. M. Janopaul, *Hospitalization and Discharge of the Mentally Ill* (Chicago: University of Chicago Press, 1968), 33.
9. Ibid.
10. M. S. Moore, "Some Myths about 'Mental Illness,'" *Archives of General Psychiatry* 32(December 1975): 1496.
11. R. Macklin, "Refusal of Psychiatric Treatment: Autonomy, Competence, and Paternalism," in *Psychiatry and Ethics*, ed. R. Edwards (Buffalo: Prometheus Books, 1982), 333.
12. Ibid., 340.
13. Ibid., 339-40.
14. "$21 Million Halcion Civil Suit Is Settled," *Psychiatric Times* 8 (17 October 1991).
15. Ibid.
16. T. C. Schelling, *Choice and Consequence* (Cambridge: Harvard University Press, 1984).
17. See, T. S. Szasz, *Ideology and Insanity: Essays on the Psychiatric Dehumanization of Man* (1970; reprint, Syracuse: Syracuse University Press, 1991), esp. Chapter 4.
18. W. Shakespeare, *Macbeth*, 5.3. 39-42.
19. See, T. S. Szasz, *The Myth of Psychotherapy*.
20. I. Batchelor, *Henderson and Gillespie's Textbook of Psychiatry*, 10th ed. (London: Oxford University Press, 1969), 544.
21. See, T. S. Szasz, *Psychiatric Justice* (1965; reprint, Syracuse: Syracuse University Press, 1988).
22. W. Blackstone, *Commentaries on the Laws of England* [1759], cited in, J. Robitscher, *The Powers of Psychiatry* (Boston: Houghton Mifflin, 1980), 25.
23. T. S. Szasz, *Psychiatric Justice*, 85-245.
24. *Jackson v. Indiana*, 406 U.S. 715 (1972).
25. W. Blackstone, *Commentaries on the Laws of England* (1759; reprint, Chicago: Callaghan and Cockcroft, 1871), vol. 2, book 4, chap. 2, p. 18.
26. See, T. S. Szasz, *Schizophrenia: The Sacred Symbol of Psychiatry* (1976; reprint, Syracuse: Syracuse University Press, 1988); and *Psychiatric Slavery: When Confinement and Coercion Masquerade as Cure* (New York: Free Press, 1977).
27. See, T. S. Szasz, *Insanity*.

Chapter 7. The Illusion of Mental Patients' Rights

1. See, I. E. Daes, *Draft Body of Principles and Guidelines for the Protection of the Mentally Ill* (Geneva: UN Commission of Human Rights, 1983).
2. New York State Commission on Quality Care for the Mentally Disabled, "Protection & Advocacy for Mentally Ill Individuals," pamphlet, n. d. (99 Washington Avenue, Albany, NY 12210). Mandated by New York State law, patients treated in medical hospitals now also receive a similarly fatuous pamphlet. See, for example, "Your Rights as a Patient" (Syracuse: State University of New York Health Science Center, University Hospital, n.d. [1991]).
3. C. Heginbotham, "The Rights of Mentally Ill People," The Minority Rights Group Report No. 74 (London: Minority Rights Group, Ltd., 1987), 3, emphasis added.
4. Ibid.
5. Ibid., 4.
6. Ibid., 5.
7. Ibid., 3.
8. B. Keller, "Mental Patients in Soviet Get New Rights," *New York Times*, 5 January 1988, pp. A1 & A11.
9. Ibid.
10. S. Grigoryants, "Soviet Psychiatric Prisoners," *New York Times*, 23 February 1988, p. A31, emphasis added.
11. Ibid.
12. T. S. Szasz, "Soviet Psychiatry: The Historical Background" [1977], in, *The Therapeutic State: Psychiatry in the Mirror of Current Events* (Buffalo: Prometheus Books, 1984), 214–18.
13. B. Keller, "Soviet Closes a Magazine Extolling Openness," *New York Times*, 19 May 1988, p. A13.
14. J. J. Rousseau, *The Social Contract* [1762], in *The Social Contract and Discourses*, trans. C. D. H. Cole (New York: Sutton, 1950), 12.
15. See Szasz, *Psychiatric Slavery*.
16. Saint T. Aquinas, *The Summa Theologica of St. Thomas Aquinas*, 2d ed., literally trans. Fathers of the English Dominican Province (London: R. T. Washbourne, 1918), 209.
17. F. J. Cornell, "Double Effect, Principle of," in, *New Catholic Encyclopedia* (New York: McGraw-Hill, 1967), 4:1020–22.
18. D. H. Smith, "On Paul Ramsey: A Covenant-Centered Ethic for Medicine," *Second Opinion* 6 (November 1987):108.
19. Ibid., 15.
20. Ibid.
21. L. Marcos, quoted in J. Barbanel, "Woman in Suit Agrees to Stay at Residence," *New York Times*, 24 November 1987, pp. B1 & B3, and, "New York Launches Effort to Remove Mentally Ill from Streets," *Psychiatric News* 23 (15 January 1988): 32.
22. A. France, quoted in B. Stevenson, ed., *The Macmillan Book of Proverbs, Maxims and Famous Phrases* (New York: Macmillan, 1948), 1364.
23. J. Barbanel, "Psychiatric Test Is Ordered for Homeless Woman," *New York Times*, 14 January 1988, p. B3.
24. Ibid.

25. J. J. Haber, "The Pitfalls of Deinstitutionalization," *R.P.C. Medical Staff—The Bulletin* (October-November-December 1987):2.
26. Ibid.
27. S. L. Rachlin, quoted in "Psychiatric Patients' Refusal to Take Their Medication Most Often Reflection of Illness," *Clinical Psychiatry News* 11 January:1.
28. Ibid.
29. Ibid.
30. Ibid.
31. Ibid., 18.
32. R. Pilon, *Human Rights and Politico-Economic Systems*, Cato's Letter #4 (Washington, D.C.: Cato Institute, 1988), 5–6.
33. T. W. Harding, "Japan's Search for International Gidelines on Rights of Mental Patients," *The Lancet* 1 (1987):677.
34. In this connection, see Szasz, *Psychiatric Slavery*, esp. 109–32.
35. See, Szasz, *Insanity* 279–366.
36. M. Roth, "Schizophrenia and the Theories of Thomas Szasz," *British Journal of Psychiatry* 129(October 1976): 326; reprinted in A. Kerr, and P. Smith, eds., *Contemporary Issues in Schizophrenia* (London: Gaskell, 1986), 114.
37. Ibid.
38. This subject was discussed in chapter 6.

Chapter 8. The Illusion of Drug Abuse Treatment

1. M. D. Anglin, and Y. Hser, "Legal Coercion and Drug Abuse Treatment: Research Findings and Social Policy Implications," in *Handbook of Drug Control in the United States*, ed. J. A. Inciardi, and J. R. Biden, Jr. (Westport, Conn.: Greenwood Press, 1990), 152.
2. F. Bastiat, *Economic Sophisms* [1845/1848], trans. Arthur Goddard (Princeton: Van Nostrand, 1964), 125–126.
3. L. Jones, "Evaluation of Drug Treatment Research Urged," *American Medical News*, 26 October 1990, 4.
4. H. D. Kleber, quoted in H. Fishman, "Whatever Happened to the War on Drugs?" *Psychiatric Times* 8(May 1991):44–45.
5. Ibid., 45.

Chapter 9. The Case Against Suicide Prevention

1. See generally, H. R. Fedden, *Suicide: A Social and Historical Study* (London: Peter Davies, 1938), and S. E. Sprott, *The English Debate on Suicide: From Donne to Hume* (Lasalle, Il: Open Court, 1961).
2. W. Blackstone, *Commentaries on the Laws of England: Of Public Wrongs* (1755–1765; reprint, Boston: Beacon Press, 1962), 212.
3. T. S. Szasz, *Insanity*, esp. 281–96.
4. S. F. Yolles, "The Tragedy of Suicide in the United States," in *Symposium on Suicide*, ed. L. Yochelson (Washington, D. C.: George Washington University, 1967), 16–17.
5. O. L. Warren, *Negligence in New York Courts*, vol. 2C (New York: Matthew Bender, 1978), 729–52.

6. H. C. Black, *Black's Law Dictionary* (St. Paul, Minn.: West, 1968), 595.
7. T. S. Szasz, "The Ethics of Suicide," in *The Theology of Medicine* (1971; reprint, Syracuse, N. Y.: Syracuse University Press, 1988), 68–85.
8. A. Artaud, "Van Gogh, the Man Suicided by Society" [1947], in A. Artaud, *Selected Writings*, ed. Susan Sontag, trans. Helen Weaver (New York: Farrar, Straus & Giroux, 1976), 496–97.
9. See chapter 10.
10. See, E. Bean, "Cigarettes and Cancer: Lawyers in U.S. Gird to Battle Tobacco Firms on Liability," *Wall Street Journal*, 1 May 1985, p. 1; and D. Margolick, "Antismoking is Encouraging Suits Against the Tobacco Industry," *New York Times*, 15 March 1985, p. 15.
11. See chapter 6.
12. In this connection, see Szasz, *Our Right to Drugs*, 150–14.

Chapter 10. The Psychiatric Will

1. T. S. Szasz, "Involuntary Mental Hospitalization: A Crime Against Humanity" [1968], in *Ideology and Insanity* 113–139.
2. T. G. Gutheil, and P. S. Applebaum, "Substituted Judgment and the Physician's Ethical Dilemma: With Special Reference to the Problem of the Psychiatric Patient," *Journal of Clinical Psychiatry* 41 (1980); 304.
3. Szasz, *The Myth of Mental Illness* and *The Myth of Psychotherapy*.
4. P. Chodoff, "The Case for Involuntary Hospitalization of the Mentally Ill," *American Journal of Psychiatry* 133(May 1976):496.
5. T. S. Szasz, *Law, Liberty, and Psychiatry: An Inquiry Into the Social Uses of Mental Health Practices* (1963; reprint, Syracuse: Syracuse University Press, 1989), and *Psychiatric Slavery*.
6. A. A. Dershowitz, "Dangerousness as a Criterion for Confinement," *Bulletin of the American Academy of Psychiatry and Law* 2(1974):172–79.
7. *O'Connor v. Donaldson*, 422 U.S. 563 (1975); p. 576, emphasis added.
8. *Rogers v. Okin*, Civil Action, 75–1610 (D. Mass. 1975).
9. J. Tauro, quoted in T. G. Gutheil, "In Search of True Freedom: Drug Refusal, Involuntary Medication, and 'Rotting with Your Rights On,'" *American Journal of Psychiatry* 137(April 1980); 328.
10. T. G. Gutheil, ibid.
11. "Patient's Right to Receive Adequate Care Explored," *Psychiatric News*, 5 December 1980, p. 1, emphasis added.
12. R. Peele, and R. Keisling, quoted in ibid., 28.
13. Ibid., emphasis added.
14. T. S. Szasz, "Your Last Will and Your Free Will," *The Alternative*, November 1974, pp. 10–11.
15. P. J. Riffolo, "The Living Will," *Journal of Family Practice* 6(1978)881–85, and R. M. Veatch, *Death, Dying, and the Biological Revolution: Our Last Quest for Responsibility* (New Haven, Conn.: Yale University Press, 1976).
16. *Natanson v. Kline*, 186 Kan. 393, 406–07, 350 P.2d., 1093 (1960), p. 1104 (dictum), cited with approval in *Woods v. Brumlop*, 71 N.M. 221, 227, 377 P.2d. 520, (1962), p. 524 (dictum), emphasis added.
17. R. M. Byrn, "Compulsory Lifesaving Treatment for the Competent Adult," *Fordham Law Review* 44(1975); 33.

18. J. W. Foley, and T. J. McGinn, "Jehovah's Witnesses and the Question of Blood Transfusion," *Postgraduate Medicine* 53(1973): 109–13.
19. *Olmstead v. United States*, 277 U.S. 438 (1928), p. 479.
20. *Application of President and Directors of Georgetown College*, 331 F. 2nd, 1010 (D.C. Cir. 1964); emphasis in original.
21. See, P. E. Raber, "Ethical and Legal Problems of the Living Will," *Geriatrics* 35(1980): 27–30.
22. Raber, "Ethical and Legal Problems," 30.
23. M. Lappe, "Dying While Living: A Critique of Allowing-to-Die Legislation," *Journal of Medical Ethics* 4(1978):196, emphasis added.
24. See, Szasz, *The Therapeutic State*.
25. "Habeas corpus," *Journal of the Libertarian Alliance* 1(1980):18.
26. See, G. J. Alexander, and T. S. Szasz, "From Contract to Status Via Psychiatry," *Santa Clara Lawyer* 13(Spring 1973):537–59.

Chapter 11. *Ex Parte* Psychiatry

1. A. de Jonge, *The Life and Times of Grigorii Rasputin* (New York: Coward, McCann & Geoghegan, 1982), 238.
2. See, for example, K. A. Wittfogel, *Oriental Despotism: A Comparative Study of Total Power* (New Haven: Yale University Press, 1957), and T. Szamuely, *The Russian Tradition*, ed. R. Conquest, (New York: McGraw-Hill, 1974).
3. See Szasz, *Insanity*, esp. chapters 9–11.
4. *The Queen Against Daniel McNaughton*, in *Daniel McNaughton: His Trial and the Aftermath*, ed. D. J. West and A. Walk (1843; reprint, London: Gaskell, 1977), 12–73.
5. Ibid., 12–13.
6. Ibid., 22.
7. Ibid., 29.
8. R. Smith, *Trial by Medicine: Insanity and Responsibility in Victorian Trials* (Edinburgh: Edinburgh University Press, 1981), 103, emphasis added.
9. *The Queen Against Daniel McNaughton*, 72.
10. Ibid., 73.
11. Black, *Black's Law Dictionary*, 661–62, emphasis added.
12. Smith, *Trial by Medicine*, 23.
13. Ibid., 31.
14. Ibid., 23.
15. S. Minor-Harper, and C. A. Innes, "Time Served in Prison and on Parole, 1984." *Bureau of Justice Statistics Special Report*, December 1987 (Washington, D.C.: U.S. Bureau of Justice) 1.
16. See, for example, "Notes and News: Human Rights Abuse in Mental Hospitals," *The Lancet*, 23 April 1988, 953–54.

Epilogue

1. R. A. Spears, *Slang and Euphemism: A Dictionary of Oaths, Curses, Insults, Sexual Slang and Metaphor, Racial Slurs, Drug Talk, Homosexual Lingo, and Related Matters* (Middle Village, N.Y.: Jonathan David Publishers, 1981), vii.

2. Ibid.
3. Ibid., ix, emphasis added.
4. Ibid.
5. T. Jefferson, "Notes on the State of Virginia" [1781], in *The Life and Selected Writings of Thomas Jefferson*, ed. A. Koch, and W. Peden (New York: Modern Library, 1944), 276.

Index

Abortion, 38, 133, 150, 156
Addiction, 5, 35. *See also* Drug abuse
African-Americans. *See* Negroes
AIDS (Acquired Immune Deficiency Syndrome), 35, 38, 143
Alcohol (alcoholism), 5-7, 81-82. *See also* Prohibition
American Bar Foundation, 115
American Civil Liberties Union. *See* New York Civil Liberties Union
American Handbook of Psychiatry (Arieti and Brody, eds.) 24
American Heritage Illustrated Encyclopedic Dictionary, 24
American Journal of Psychiatry, 4, 163
American Psychiatric Association (APA), 2, 35
Americans With Disabilities Act (AWDA), 4-5
Aquinas, Thomas, Saint, 132-133
Artaud, Antonin, 153
Association of Medical Officers of Asylums (British), 2
Association for Retarded Citizens (ARC), 39

Barnum, P. T., 38
Bastiat, Frederic, 145
Batchelor, Ivor, 118
Behavior, distinguished from disease, 1, 21-22, 30-35
Beheading, of drug dealers, 145
Bennett, William, 145
Bible, 24-25, 35
Biden, Joseph, 144
Birth control. *See* Contraception
Black's Law Dictionary, 150
Blackstone, William, 119, 122, 149
Blasphemy, 102
Bleuler, Eugen, 22, 26
Brandeis, Louis, 167 , 172
Broadmoor Hospital, 179
Brown, Joyce, 135-137
Burch, Darrell, 113-115

Burger, Warren, 167
Burke, Edmund, 135
Bush, George, 146

Calvin, John, 46
Casares, Adolfo Bioy, 101
Cellular Pathology (Virchow), 22
Charcot, Jean-Martin, 104, 105
Chesterton, Gilbert K., 111
Choice and Consequence (Schelling), 117
Civil commitment. *See* Mental hospitalization, involuntary
Civil liberties. *See* Rights
Coercion, and psychiatry. *See* Mental hospitalization, involuntary
Commitment, civil. *See* Mental hospitalization, involuntary
Competence. *See* Incompetence
Communism. *See* Marxism
Constitution, of the United States, 102, 121, 162, 167
Contraception, 134, 156, 157
Contract, 111, 118, 123-126,
Copernicus, Mikolaj, 108
Crime, and mental illness. *See* Mental illness
Criminal trial, and psychiatry. *See* Ex parte psychiatry

Darwin, Charles, 108
Deinstitutionalization, 130
Delirium. *See* Mental incompetence
Deviance, dictionaries of, 37-97
Diagnosis, by consensus groups, 9
distinguished from disease, 5-9
Diagnostic and Statistical Manual (APA), various version of, 1, 9, 37
Diagnostic and Statistical Manual, DSM-III (APA), 4, 32-33, 37
Diagnostic and Statistical Manual, DSM-III-R (APA), 4, 33, 36, 37-45

Diagnostic and Statistical Manual,
    DSM-IV (APA), 7, 37
Dictionary of American Slang (Went-
    worth and Flexner), 91
Dictionary of the History of Ideas (Wie-
    ner, ed.), 28
Disease, distinguished from behavior, 1,
    21–22, 30–35
Don Quixote, 103
Donaldson case. *See O'Connor v.*
    Donaldson (1975)
Double effect, principle of, 132–135
Drinkers Dictionary, The (Franklin), 81,
    83–88
Drug abuse,
    illusion of drug abuse treatment, 143–
    146
Drunkenness,
    contemporary dictionary of, 91–97,
    dictionaries of/synonyms for, 81–97,
    and driving, 6–7, *See also* Alcohol
DSM-IV Options Book (APA), 37

Eskimos, language of, 24, 28
Ex parte psychiatry, 173–181

Farnham, William, 13
Finnegan's Wake (Joyce), 23
First Amendment, to the U.S. Constitu-
    tion, 102
Fliess, Wilhelm, 105
Foster, Jody, 7
France, Anatole, 28, 135
Frances, Allen, 7
Franklin, Benjamin, 81, 83–84
Freud, Sigmund, 2, 13, 19, 34, 103–109,
    118,
Freud, Sophie, 22
Furor diagnosticus, 37

Gardner, Jim, 39
Glossolalia,
    compared with schizophrenic (psy-
    chotic) speech, 23–25
    and Holy Spirit, 23–25
Grigoryants, Sergei, 131
Guillotine, Joseph, 145
Gusyeva, Chionya, 173–174

Halcion, 117

Haldol, 136–137
Hamlet (Shakespeare), 13–19
Handbook of Drug Control in the United
    States (Inciardi and Biden), 144
Harding, Timothy W., 139
Heginbotham, Chris, 129–130
Henderson and Gillespie's Textbook of
    Psychiatry (Batchelor), 118–119
Hinckley, John W., Jr., 7, 180
Holmes, Oliver Wendell, Jr., 102
Holy Spirit, and glossolalia, 23–25
Homosexuality, 35, 38
Human Action (Mises), 158–159
Hutchings Psychiatric Center (Syra-
    cuse), renaming of, 78

Inciardi, James, 144
Incompetence. *See* Mental incompetence
Insanity. *See also*, Incompetence, Irratio-
    nality, Mental illness,
Inquisition, and doctors, 144
Involuntary mental hospitalization. *See*
    Mental hospitalization

Jefferson, Thomas, 83, 103, 185
Jehovah's Witnesses, and right to refuse
    treatment, 123–124, 167
Jesus, 102, 175
Joyce, James, writing diagnosed as
    schizophrenic, 23
Jung, Carl, 118

Kant, Immanuel, 159
Kaplan, Harold I., 24
Keywords (Williams), 28
Kleber, Herbert D., 146
Kleptomania. *See* Shoplifting
Knock (Romains), 183
Kraepelin, Emil, 114
Kraus, Karl, 22, 106

Larson, Cedric, 83
Last will, 165
Leff, Julian, 22–23
"Lexicon of Prohibition" (Wilson), 82,
    89–90
Lincoln, Abraham, 33
Living will, 166
Locke, John, 122

Lourdes, cures as compared with psychoanalysis, 105

Macbeth (Shakespeare), 18–19, 118
Macklin, Ruth, 116–117
Mahon, Maeve, 136
Malpractice, and suicide, 150–152
Marcos, Imelda, 5
Marcos, Luis, 135–136
Martin, J. R., 26
Marx, Karl, 2
  and Freud, 107–109
Medicaid, 8
Medicare, 8
Mellaril, 138
Mencken, Henry L., 29, 78, 81, 82
Menninger, Karl, 37
Menninger, William, 37
Mens rea, 122
Mental hospitalization,
  involuntary, 112–117, 134–141, 144
Mental hospital, synonyms for, 78–79
Mental illness,
  as brain disease, 1–3, 13, 25–27, 30–31,
  and crime, 173–181,
  synonyms for, 46–77. *See also* Mental incompetence
Mental incompetence, 111–126 , 149,
  delirium as, 120–121
Mental patients, illusion of rights of, 127–141
Methadone, 143
McNaughton, Daniel, trial of, 177–180
Mill, John Stuart, 147
Moore, Michael, 115–116
Moses, 35
Moses of Michelangelo, The (Freud), 13
Myth of Mental Illness, The (Szasz), 21

Nash, Ogden, 91
Natanson v. Kline, 166
National Association for Mental Health (UK), 129
Nazi doctors, as agents of the state, 144
Negligence, professional. *See* Malpractice
Negroes, renaming of, 39, 82
New Catholic Encyclopedia, 24

New York Civil Liberties Union, and involuntary mental hospitalization, 135–137
New York State Commission on Quality Care for the Mentally Disabled, 128
Nietzsche, Friedrich, 185
Non compos mentis. See Mental incompetence

O'Connor v. Donaldson (1975), 161
Onassis, Jacqueline Kennedy, 5
On Liberty (Mill), 147
Orthodoxy (Chesterton), 111

Parens patriae, principle of and psychiatry, 161, 168
Paternalism, 159
Pennsylvania Gazette, 83
Peel, Sir Robert, 177
Picasso, Pablo, 26
Pilon, Roger, 138–139
Polanyi, Michael, 3
Pollock, Jackson, 26
Poor Richard's Almanack (Franklin), 83, 85
Postman, Neil, 33
Pound, Ezra, 119, 121
Presumption, of incompetence/irrationality, 112, 115, 117
  of innocence/guilt, 111
  of insanity/mental illness, 115, 117
Prohibition, 81, 89
Psychiatric News (APA), 7, 163
Psychiatric will, 159–172
Psychiatry, and/as religion, 101–110, 138
"Psychical (or Mental) Treatment" (Freud), 2
Psychoanalysis, 2,
  and religion, 103–110
Psychopathology of Everyday Life, The (Freud), 34

Rachlin, Stephen L., 137
Ramsey, Paul, 133
Randolph, Thomas Jefferson, 103
Rasputin, Grigorii, 173
Reagan, Ronald, 7
Religion, 1–2,
  opiate of the people (Marx), 2

and psychiatry, 101–110
and psychoanalysis, 103–110
Right to die, 168
Rights, of mental patients, illusion of, 127–141
to refuse medication, 128, 137–138
"Rights of Mentally Ill People" (Heginbotham), 129–130
Rochester, Sherry, 26
Rogers, Will, 4, 89
Romains, Jules, 183
Roth, Sir Martin, 25, 140
Rousseau, Jean Jacques, 132
Rubinow, David, 7
Rushdie, Salman, 101

Sadock, Benjamin J., 24
Schelling, Thomas C., 117
Schizophrenese. *See* Schizophrenia
Schizophrenia, 2, 25, 127,
and language, 22–27
compared to glossolalia, 23–25
"Schizovisia," 25
Science, v. scientism, 3
Scott, Sir Walter, 22
Second Part of King Henry the Fourth (Shakespeare)
Self defense, killing in, 132–133
Sex, addiction, 35
Shakespeare, William, 13–19, 81, 117, 118
Shoplifting, 4–6
as addiction, 5
Smith, David, 133
Smythies, J. R., 23
Soviet Union, and psychiatry, 130–131
Freud on, 107,
renaming of cities, 38
Speaking in tongues. *See* Glossolalia
Spears, Richard A., 183–184

Strachey, James, 34
Suicide, case against prevention, 147–158,
compared with contraception, 157
Summa Theologica (Aquinas), 132–133
Supreme Court (U.S.), 36, 113–115, 121, 161

Tarsis, Valeriy, 78n
Tauro, Joseph, 162–163
Ten Commandments, 35
Theological state (society), 1
Therapeutic state (society), 1, 170–171
Therapy by the judiciary, 137
Twain, Mark, v

United Nations, and mental patients' rights, 127
USSR. *See* Soviet Union

Virchow, Rudolf, 22
Voltaire, 139

War on Drugs, 144–146
Ward 7 (Tarsis), 78
Webster's Third New International Dictionary, 24, 29, 38
Wilson, Edmund, 82, 89
Winick, Bruce J., 114
Winslow, Forbes, 180
Wittgenstein, Ludwig, 22, 33,
writing diagnosed as schizophrenic, 23
World Federation for Mental Health, 129
World Health Organization, 21, 129–130, 143

Yolles, Stanley, 149

Zinermon v. Burch (1990), 113–115